Grand Priory of the Maltese Islands
Military and Hospitaller Order of St Lazarus of Jerusalem

Leprosy Archives - Maltese Islands

Compiled and Edited by
Charles Savona-Ventura

2021

© Charles Savona-Ventura 2021

All rights reserved. No part of this publication may be reproduced, stored in a retrieval system or transmitted in any form or by any means, electronic, mechanical, photocopying, recording or otherwise without the prior permission of the publisher.

Published by
Raoul Follereau Foundation – Order of Charity [V/O 0980]
Grand Priory of the Maltese Islands
Military and Hospitaller Order of St Lazarus of Jerusalem
Malta

Printed by
Lulu Press Inc.
Morrisville,
North Carolina,
U.S.A.

1st edition [2006] *published by*
Grand Priory of the Maltese Islands
Military and Hospitaller Order of St Lazarus of Jerusalem
Malta

ISBN: 978-1-6780-9605-2

Contents

History of Leprosy in Malta 5

Biography: Prominent Maltese leprologists 17

Maltese Leprosaria 23

Support Organizations in Malta 29

Prevalence, Incidence & Hospital Statistics 37

Annotated Bibliography 45

Maltese Legislation 115

History of Leprosy in Malta

Introduction [1]

Leprosy also known as Hansen's disease, is a chronic granulomatous disease caused by the bacterium Mycobacterium leprae and affecting the peripheral nerves and mucosa of the upper respiratory tract; skin lesions are the primary external symptom. Left untreated, leprosy can be progressive, causing permanent damage to the skin, nerves, limbs, and eyes. The disease has a long history in the Mediterranean Basin with the first clinical description being possibly that of the 16th century BC Ebers Papyrus. Archaeological evidence confirms the presence of the disease in Egypt during the 2nd century BC. The disease was subsequently spread throughout the Mediterranean. The first accurate description of the disease was written by the Greek physician Galen of Pergamun in 150 AD.

There is no evidence to date of the presence of the disease in the archaeological record of the Maltese Islands. Similarly, the few scanty Classical texts make no reference to the infection. Based on linguistics, the disease in Malta probably has very ancient origins. The Maltese vernacular term for leprosy is *Ġdiem* [leper = *mġiddem*]; a word that originates from the Arabic جُذَام = *jozam* [leper = مجذوم = *majzoon*]. The Maltese Islamic influence is known to have lasted from 870-1249 AD. In 1240, Muslims accounted for about 40% of the Maltese population. Islamic society looked upon leprosy as a punishment from God for immorality, and the Maliki law allowed either partner to dissolve a marriage on the basis of leprosy. Lepers were not allowed to mix with the rest of the healthy community. In a *hadith* (traditions of the Prophet Muhammad) the Prophet is reported as saying: *wa-firr min al-majdhumin kama tafirru min al-asad* (Flee from the leper as you flee from the lion); while in another *hadith* we find the Prophet unwilling to meet a leper who, when calling on him to pledge his *bay'a* (oath of allegiance), was asked to stay away and was told his *bay'a* was accepted. The 13th century *Geniza* writings record the testimony of Abu al-Tahir b. al-Husayn: 'In the name of God the Compassionate, the merciful. Those who set their hand hereto and have fully declared their names, among those men in positions of trust whose word in their attestations is accepted, hereby attest that they attended Ibrahim al-Yahudi, who has been <u>affected by such black bile as has caused him to develop leprosy</u>, and that fact is such that <u>it debars him from mixing freely with the Muslims and from earning his living</u>. Having ascertained the truth of the matter by their having attended and established an accurate diagnosis of his illness, and, having been requested to issue an attestation of their finding, they have complied with the request, such attestation being issued on the first day of Rabi` al-Akhir of the year six hundred and sixty [23 February AD 1262]. Testimony: I attended the above named and The Am-in All ... in him, which is his found him to be suffering from illness leprosy. <u>He may not mix freely with the Muslims because that condition is a</u>

---

[1] Originally published in the *Malta Medical Journal* Volume 20 Issue 04 December 2008 p. 34-38 – under the authorship of George G. Buttigieg, Charles Savona-Ventura, Kyril Micallef Stafrace. Further annotated with data published in Savona-Ventura C. Hansen's Disease in Malta. *The Sunday Times (Malta)*, 29th January 1995, 32-33 and other sources.

transmissible and communicable disease. Signed by Abu al-Tahir b. al-Husayn.[2] There is therefore no doubt that leprosy was present during in the Mediterranean during the Medieval Period. Frederick II formulated a set of legal constitutions in 1231. These make no specific mention to leprosy. In contrast, the Lombard King Rothari in the code of laws promulgated in the 7th century makes specific mention whereby those identified as lepers were 'expelled from the district or from his house so that her lives alone, he shall not have the right to alienate his property or give it to anyone. Because on the day that he is expelled from his home, it is as if he died. Nevertheless, while he lives he should be nourished on the income from that which remains.[3] The Crusades, initiated in 1099 in an effort to recapture the Holy Land from the Seljuk Turks, established links with the Eastern Mediterranean lands helping to further spread the infection to Southern and Central Europe. This link persisted until the expulsion of the Christian forces from Acre in 1291.

In nearby Southern Italy, Emperor Frederick II of Sicily in 1226 accepted the establishment of a *magister infirmorum Ecclesaiae S. Lazari* in Capua by the nobleman Lazaro di Raimo. By 1273, five lepers were being tended by at this hospital managed by the Order of St. Lazarus – a hospitaller and military Order that saw its origins in the Holy Land whose main brief was to care for lepers. Following Pope Clement IV's Bull of August 1265, Charles I adopted and ordered that all lepers in his domain were to be placed under government of Order of St Lazarus.[4] There is no definitive evidence that the Maltese Islands were directly influenced by these Royal edicts; however, the Islands were bound by the same laws and regulations appertaining to nearby Sicily. It has been suggested that the Medieval *hospitalis Sanctj Franciscj*, situated outside the Medieval walls of Mdina, had been initially established as a leprosarium.[5] No documentary proof has however been found to substantiate this assertion. The hospital is known to have been definitely in existence by 1372 and probably by 1299.[6] The hospital was managed by members of the Franciscan Order who included the care of lepers in their vocation. By 1494, the hospital documentation makes no mention of lepers but refers only to "*poveri abitanti*".[7]

However, leprosy had become less of a problem in Europe after the Plague epidemic of the 14th century and the lack of specific mention in the 15th century documentation does not preclude the use of the hospital facilities for lepers in earlier centuries. The first documented case of leprosy termed *erga corpore morbo lepre* is said to have affected a Gozitan woman Garita Xejbais who bequeathed land to the Church in 1492. In contrast to what had occurred in earlier centuries in Europe, where lepers were considered "the living dead"

---

[2] *Ms. T-S NS 327.51: Geniza writings*, Cambridge University Library.
[3] Skimmer P. *Health & Medicine in Early Medieval Southern Italy.* Brill, Netherlands, 1997, 59-61, 77.
[4] Savona-Ventura C. *The Hospitaller Knights of St. Lazarus.* Grand Priory of the Maltese Islands – MHOSLJ, Malta, 2006
[5] Gulia G. Sopra un caso de Lebbra dei Greci. Il Barth, 29 January 1874, 3(19):372-377
[6] On the 20th July – 7th August 1299, Pope Boniface VIII appoints Cardinal Bishop Gerardus of Sabina as an Apostolic Legate to the Kingdom of Sicily [including Malta] who is authorised to grant up to a hundred days of indulgence to the faithful who assist in the building of churches and the running of hospitals. *Reg. Vat. F f.ccxlviiiii-cclii verso, ep.xxiii.* Transcribed in: Aquilina GA, Fiorini S, editors. Documentary Sources of Maltese history. Part IV Documents at the Vatican. No. 2 Archivio Segreto Vaticano: Cancellaria Apostolica and Camera Apostolica and related sources at the Biblioteca Apostolica Vaticana 416-1479. University Press, Malta, 2005, doc.41, ep. XXIII, 63-64.
[7] Savona-Ventura C. Hospitaller activities in Medieval Malta. *Malta Medical Journal*, 2007, 19:48-52

and stripped of all legal rights, the 1492 document suggests that lepers in the Maltese Islands during the 15th century retained their legal and inheritance rights.[8]

Hospitaller Period

The 16th century was to see the arrival of the hospitaller Order of St. John to the Maltese Islands. The Order was familiar with leprosy having seen and suffered from its ravages in the Holy Land. During the reign of Grandmaster Hugues de Revel (1258- 1277), the Order had established the rule that "if in any country there be a Brother who is a leper, he may not wear the Habit from that time forward, and may not come among the Brethren, but he should be provided with food and clothing".[9] The Order of St. John, in addition to hospices and charity houses, also ran leprosaria in a large number of places in Europe, albeit mostly catering for the pilgrims or travellers and the poor.[10] In Rhodes, the Order had regulated stringent public health laws to limit the spread of the disease in the *Domini Sanatatis*, promulgated during the reign of Grandmaster Emery D'Amboise (1530-1512). The "sick of Saint Lazarus" were beneficiaries of special charities from the Order and cared for in their homes. These regulations debarred infected individuals from having any social intercourse with healthy ones who in turn were prohibited under penalty of a hefty fine from receiving any goods from lepers. Furthermore, lepers were precluded from practicing certain occupations unless licensed by the sanitary authorities who ensured that material goods belonging to lepers was not physically passed on to healthy people.[11] These regulations suggest that while lepers were still considered a threat to the community, they were not considered sufficiently infective to require seclusion in designated leprosaria. When admitted to the *Sacra Infermeria*, leprous individuals were nursed in cubicles.[12] These sanitary regulations were adopted in the Maltese Islands after the arrival of the Order in 1530.

The first recorded case of leprosy in Malta during the Hospitaller Period involved a Dominican friar who died in the Rabat convent in Malta in 1630. The documents relate the purchase of a slave by the Dominican Priory during the previous year to care for the sick friar.[13] The second half of the seventeenth century saw an increasing preoccupation with the disease. The infectivity of the disease was well recognised and concerns about the fate of the sufferers were voiced by the Gran Consiglio of the Order in 1659.[14] In 1679, the *Commissione* set up to regulate the management of the hospital services proposed that lepers should be given financial aid and treated in their homes. Foreign sufferers with leprosy were to be admitted to the *Falanga* of

---

[8] Busuttil J. Fiorini S, editors. *Documentary Sources of Maltese history. Part V Documents in the Curia of the Archbishop of Malta. No. 1 The Registrum Fundationum Beneficiorum Insulae Gaudisii 1435-1545*. University Press, Malta, 2006, doc.57, 80-81
[9] King EJ. *The Rule Statutes and Customs of the Hospitallers 1099-1310, With Introductory Chapters and Notes*, Methuen & Co. Ltd., London, 1934
[10] Buttigieg GG, Micallef Stafrace K. The Order of St. John's Crusade against leprosy. *Sacra Militia*, 2008, 7:29-38
[11] National Malta Library (NML). *Manuscript 153*, fol. 421; *Manuscript 740*, fol. 36t (as reported by P. Cassar: *The Medical History of Malta*. Wellcome Historical Medical Library, London, 1965, 210).
[12] Gabriel A. *La cité de Rhodes*. Vol. 1 (1921); Vol. 2 (1923). E. de Boccard éditeur, París
[13] Archives of the Dominican Priory, Rabat (Malta). *De statu trium conventum. Parte I*, f.129t, 188 (as reported by P. Cassar, 1965, 210)
[14] NML. *Commissione perche provedesse ai poveri affetti dal terribile morbo della lebra. Liber Concilium. Archives of the Order of St. John of Malta (AOM) 121*, fol.53 (as reported by P. Cassar, 1965, 210-211).

the *Sacra Infermeria* and isolated from the other regular patients. Before admission, the patient was to be carefully examined by the hospitaller, the infirmarian and the *prud hommes* to confirm the diagnosis.[15] The *Status Animarum* of 1687 records only one 30-year-old female living at Qormi in Malta suffering from leprosy in a population of about 45288 (prevalence 2.21 per 100,000 population) with *maritus non cohabitat*. This registration confirms that lepers were managed in isolation in the community rather than designated leprosaria but living separately from her spouse.[16]

This sole record in the *Status Animarum* does not preclude the presence of other afflicted individuals, particularly since Dr. Giuseppe Zammit is reported to have in 1687 described five cases to the Academia Medica.[17] Barbers in 1702 were warned of the personal danger when attending sufferers from the disease.[18] The 1725 *Sacra Infermeria* regulations provided a daily allowance to sufferers.[19] Giuseppe Demarco further discussed this skin infection in a chapter of the treatise *Tractatus affectuum cutaneorum*.[20] Further reported cases included a nun of the Monastery of St. Catherine, Valletta who in 1770 "developed ulcers and fever and also became leprous" and subsequently succumbed to the disease; and the leprous son of Turkish official who in 1771 arrived in Malta from Turkey on his way to Marseille in search of a cure.[21]

Nineteenth century

A number of solitary cases of leprosy were described by the medical community in the early decades of the nineteenth century. In 1808, 3 cases (1 Maltese) were described by Dr. Saydon among the crew on a Turkish ship. Cases of leprosy were also discussed during the meetings of the *Accademia Medica Maltese* that functioned until 1837.[22] These probably refer to the cases described in later reports attributable to Prof. F.G. Schinas dated 1835 and to Dr. Gravagna dated 1837. During the period 1839-1858, seven cases – four males and three females – were reported to have succumbed to this infection.[23] In spite of these case reports, in 1862 in replying to a questionnaire sent by the Special Committee of the Royal College of Physicians, leprosy was stated to be non-existent on the Islands, though the possibility of the disease being present but

---

[15] NML: *AOM 262*, f.97, 141 (as reported by P. Cassar, 1965, 210-211); Bonello G. Reforms in the Holy Infirmary, 1680. *Malta Medical Journal*. 2007; 19:45-49.
[16] Fiorini S. Status Animarum II: A Census of 1687. *Proceedings of History Week 1984* (Fiorini S, editor), University Press, Malta, 1986, 41-100
[17] *Reports on leprosy in Malta by a Committee appointed by H.E. the governor in 1917 – Final report*. Government Printing Office, Malta, 1919
[18] Galea J, Bonnici E. Leprosy in Malta. *Leprosy Review*, 1957, 28: 140
[19] *Notizia della Sacra Infermeria e della carica delli Commissarj delle Povere Inferme*. R. Bernaba, Rome, 1725 (English translation: E.E. Hume. *Medical work of the Knight Hospitallers of Saint John of Jerusalem*. John Hopkins Press, Baltimore, 1940, 137-148)
[20] Demarco G. Tractatus affectuum cutaneorum. NML Ms. 36, 1764, n.p.
[21] NML. Manuscript 1146 bis, f.74, 189.
[22] *Reports on leprosy….., 1919, op. cit.*
[23] Gulia, 1874, *op. cit.*; Sammut I. Le Lebbre dei Greci. *Il Barth*, 4 April 1874, 3(20):399-400

unidentified was accepted.[24] By 1874, Malta included among the seats of leprosy, though noted to be "not commonly encountered".[25] Further cases were reported by Dr. G. Gulia and Dr. I. Sammut.[26]

The latter half of the nineteenth century saw a marked increase in the number of affected cases probably resulting from increasing contact with North Africa through returning migrants, refugees, and increased shipping. The stationing of a large detachment of Indian Troops at Imriehel in Malta in 1878 may also have been contributory since the earliest statistics of origin of leprosy cases showed that the majority of local lepers came from villages in the vicinity.[27] The gradual and steady increase in the number of leprosy cases stimulated the authorities to appoint in 1883 a committee composed of seven doctors to investigate the epidemiology of the disease and suggest methods of control. The main result of the Committee's work after examining 30 cases was the decision to introduce compulsory segregation, even though they believed that the disease was hereditary rather than contagious.[28] A population survey was conducted in 1890 to assess the size of the problem. Only 69 known cases of leprosy were identified suggesting a prevalence rate of 42 per 100,000 population; eight of which lived in Gozo – four from Nadur. Only eleven cases were in an advanced stage of the disease and had admitted themselves to the Asylum for the Aged and Incurables, commonly known as the Poor House. The greater number of cases in Malta came from rural areas, mainly Qormi and Mosta. Only one came from Valletta.[29]

Twentieth century

As a result of the 1883 committee's report, the Council of Government in 1893 issued the Lepers Ordinance No. VII entitled An Ordinance for checking the spread of the disease commonly known as Leprosy. The ordinance provided for the compulsory notification under pain of legal penalties of every case of leprosy immediately it was recognised. Cases confirmed by the newly established Leprosy Board, composed of five doctors, were to be immediately segregated in a Leprosarium for as long as they were deemed a public danger. An *ad hoc* Leprosarium was constructed near the Poor House, the male section being occupied in 1890, while females were admitted after 1912.[30] The female wing of the Leper Hospital was completed in April 1911 and the new chapel of the hospital was blessed by the Vicar-General on the 1st October 1911. The building consisted of a central block with a main entrance hall leading to the administration's offices, a chapel, the residential quarters of the three nursing Sisters of Charity and the chaplain, the dispensary, stores, kitchen, and laundry. On either side of the entrance hall were two wings – one for males and one for women. The wards accommodated a total of 90 male and 70 female patients. The total hospital male and female population

---

[24] Report on Leprosy by the Royal College of Physicians prepared for Her Majesty's Secretary of State for the Colonies, with an Appendix. London, 1867. *Il Barth*, 6 August 1874, 3(21-22):424-427.
[25] Contagiosita` della elefantiasi dei Greci. *Il Barth*, 6 August 1874, 3(21-22):442.
[26] Gulia, 1874, *op. cit.*; Sammut, 1874, *op. cit.*
[27] Bugeja J. Leprosy in Malta. *Reports on the working of Government departments during the financial year 1930-31*. Government Printing Office, Malta, 1932, Section R:17-30
[28] *Reports on leprosy….*, 1919, *op. cit.*
[29] Medical & Health Archives: *Letters to Government from 20 April 1888 to 8 April 1895*. f.300 (as reported in P. Cassar, 1965, 213)
[30] Galea & Bonnici, 1957, *op. cit.*

in 1911 however amounted to 73 inmates.[31] The hospital population reached its high-water mark in 1917 with 114 inmates (71 males; 43 females); suggesting a prevalence rate of 49 per 100,000 population. The disease thereafter showed a progressive decline (Figure 1).[32]

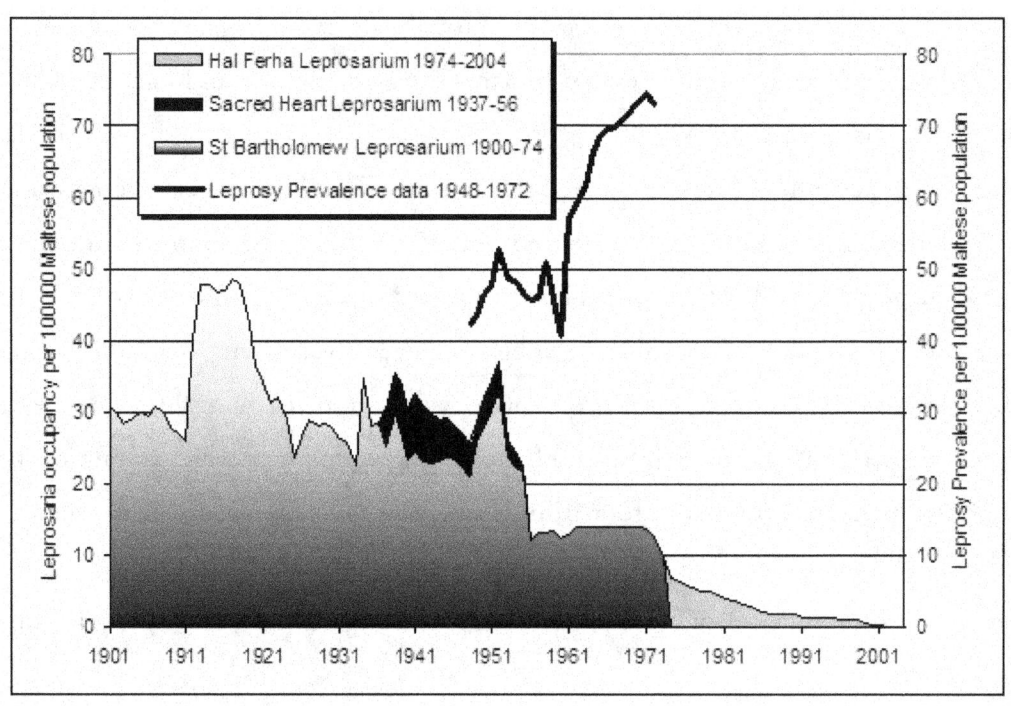

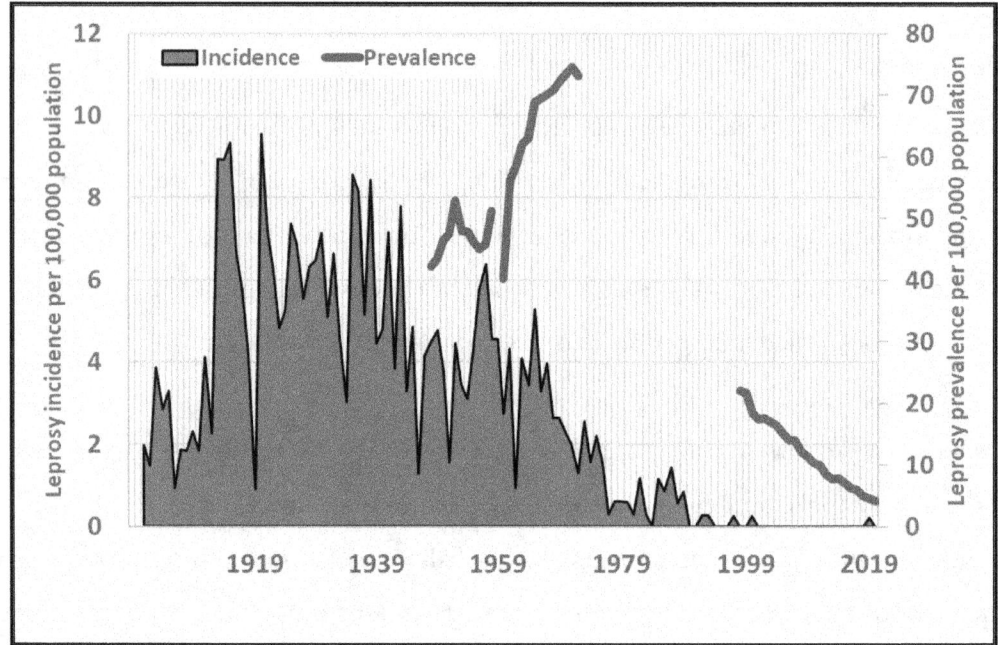

Figure 1: Hospital Leper Population and Incidence – Prevalence rates 1901-2005
[Source: Annual Reports of the Department of Health]

Concurrently with the opening of the Leper Asylum, special regulations were issued to ensure and maintain complete segregation from the outside community. The severe restrictions imposed by these

---

[31] Pace Bardon C. Office of the Comptroller of Charitable Institutions, Valletta, 28 June 1912. *Reports on the Workings of Government Department during the Financial Year 1911-12*. Government Printing Office, Malta, 1912, M2
[32] Galea A. Office of the Comptroller of Charitable Institutions, Valletta, 6 November 1923. *Reports on the Workings of Government Department during the Financial Year 1922-23*. Government Printing Office, Malta, 1925, Q1-2

regulations were greatly resented by the lepers so that the first five or six years were marked by incessant complaints, frequent disturbances, escapes from the Asylum, and attacks on the personnel. The first disturbance occurred in May 1900 - only five months after the first patients were received. Fifty-four male lepers overpowered their attendants and found their way out of the Asylum. Another disturbance occurred in September 1900. Order was restored on both occasions after intervention by the police.[33] In view of these repeat disturbances, a detachment of police was retained in the Asylum to maintain order. This detachment was removed in 1903 when the hospital attendants were given executive police powers. The lepers settled to a normal life in the hospital by 1907, though complaints continued to crop up. While the 1893 Ordinance did not allow the lepers to leave the Asylum except to visit sick family members or to emigrate abroad, individuals were granted special leave of absence for a few hours for domestic, legal or financial transaction which required their presence.

OCCUPATION	MALE	FEMALE
Agricultural labourers	81	22
Day labourers	47	-
Hawkers/shopkeepers	18	4
Stone masons	18	-
Fishermen	16	-
Carters/cabmen	16	-
Coalheavers	15	-
Servants/housemaids	6	12
Plasterers	4	-
Carpenters/blacksmiths	4	-
Soldiers/seamen	4	-
Students/clerks	4	-
Priests/nuns	2	1
Washerwomen/seamstresses	-	7
Housewives	-	27
Lacemakers/spinners/weavers	-	15
Beggars	4	2
Other/unspecified	25	18

Table 1: Occupation of hospitalized lepers during period 1900-1929
[Source: Annual Reports of the Department of Health]

By 1901 inmates were being allowed to go out accompanied two at a time for walks in the country. This was extended in 1902 to a drive in a cart, cab (after 1910) or bus (after 1930). By 1907, the inmates appeared to have accepted the restrictions.[34] In 1916, as a result of complaints regarding the food and clothing supplies, the Governor appointed a Board "to inquire into the discipline of the Leper Asylum, and to recommend efficient measures for its proper maintenance, and to ascertain whether the inmates had any substantial grounds of complaint, and to suggest the means of removing any grievances that were well

---

[33] *Letters to Government......*, 1900-02, f.515,611
[34] Bugeja, 1932, *op. cit.*

founded". The board reported that the grievances were generally unfounded and were the result of the restrictive circumstances. It also opinionated the low degree of communicability of leprosy. A second Committee was appointed in 1918 "to study de novo the question of the seclusion of lepers enforced by the law". This Committee maintained that compulsory segregation was still necessary but emphasised that patients should have the right to all the necessary comforts and the best therapeutic treatment. The Report also gave an estimated prevalence of leprosy as 47.2 per 100,000 population. As a result of this report, an amended Lepers Ordinance was published in 1919, while the hospital regulations were revised. The new regulations required internment of the leper only seven days after confirmation and allowed for the eventual discharge of the patient when the disease process was considered arrested and there remained no further risk to the public.[35]

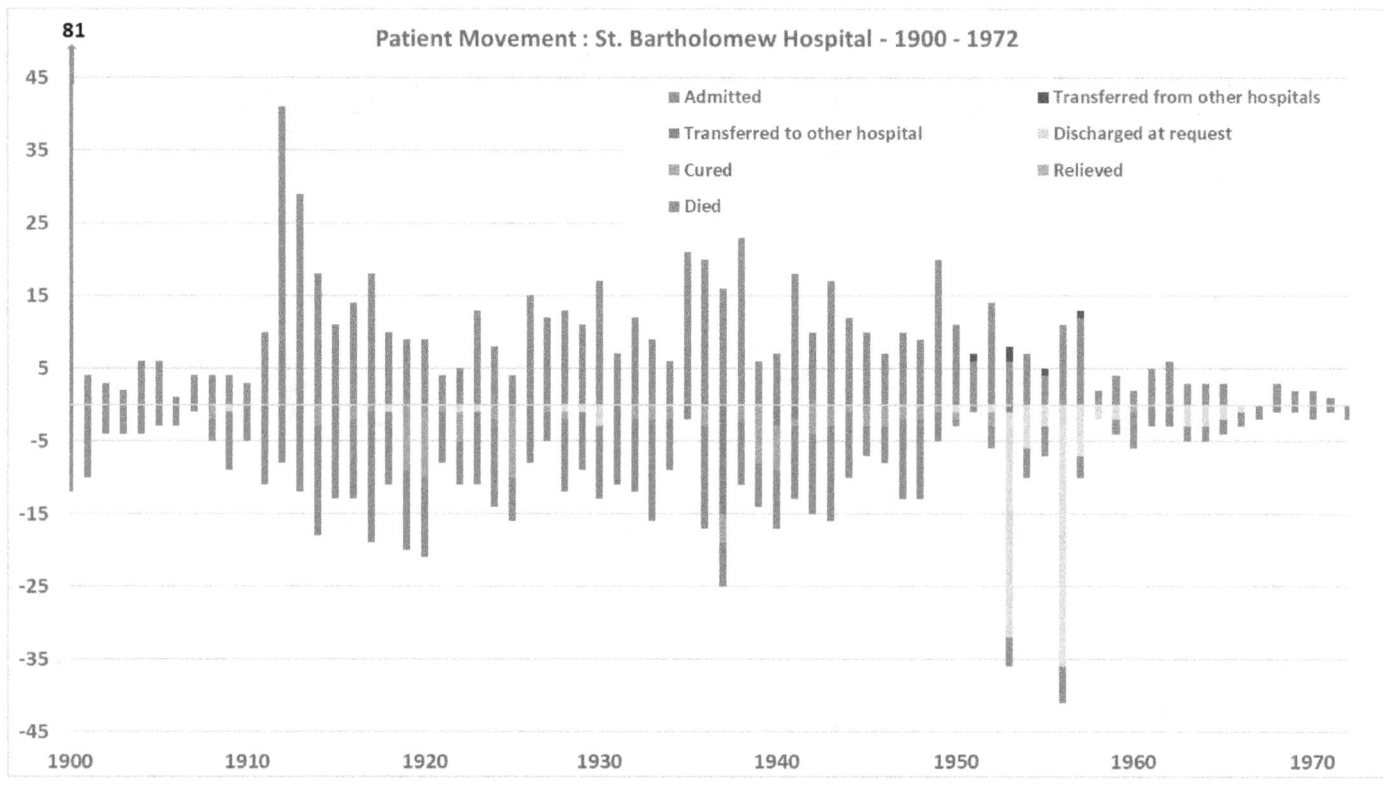

Figure 2: Admissions & Discharges from the Leprosarium 1900-1972
[Source: Annual Reports of the Department of Health]

As a result also of the 1919 Committee's recommendations, a number of innovations were instituted to alleviate the lepers' situation in the Asylum. The patients were given the facility to be usefully employed for domestic work and general maintenance in the Institution, while the surrounding grounds were given over for poultry farming and cultivation by the inmates. The increasing useful activity was well received by the inmates. Furthermore, a common room with indoor games and reading material was made available, while

---

[35] *Ordinance XX of 1919: To make provisions with respect to the disease commonly known as leprosy. The Lepers Ordinance Chapter 73 of the Revised Edition.* Eventually amended by Act. XV of 1929, Ord. XXV of 1939, Ord. XVI of 1942, and mostly repealed by Act XI of 1953. Further modified by Legal Notice 46 of 1965; Act LVIII of 1974; Legal Notice 148 of1975; Acts VIII of 1990 and V of 2007; and Legal Notice 346 of 2008.

entertainment was regularly provided. The realisation and acceptance that leprosy had a very low infectivity rate allowed the introduction after 1929 of family visits by the inmates accompanied by an attendant. During the 1930s, inmates of the leprosarium whose families resided in Gozo, generally averaging 11 males and 4 females, were transported to the Hospital for Infectious Disease in Gozo for a few days once every quarter for an aggregate period of about 29 days. During their stay, they were housed on the ground floor of the hospital.[36]

Further amendments to the Lepers Ordinance were made in 1929 to enable the examination of contacts of diagnosed cases, while a new leprosarium was opened in the old Married Quarters at Fort Chambray in Gozo in 1937. In the same period the Lepers Hospital, previously managed in conjunction with the Poor House, was given an autonomous management; while the hospitals' names were eventually changed to Saint Bartholomew Hospital (Malta) and Sacred Heart Hospital (Gozo) to remove the stigmata associated with the disease. The low infectivity of the disease was eventually accepted, and the segregation policy was removed in 1953 when compulsory internment was abolished except under special circumstances.

St. Bartholomew Hospital in 1956 was described as an old but fine and spacious building with a bed complement of 118 beds. However, during 1953-54, it only housed an average of 74 patients. The hospital had better amenities than many of the other hospitals in Malta. The wards, corridors and gardens were noted to be spacious and pleasing. There was an entertainment hall and efforts were being made to organize shows and outings for the inmates. The hospital was managed by one medical officer, the Medical Superintendent, who was relieved by one of the doctors at contiguous St Vincent de Paule Hospital on his off-days.[37] The Sacred Heart Hospital in Gozo, situated in the old Married Quarters at Fort Chambray, had a bed complement of 27 beds. Thirteen men and two women, originally from Gozo, were transferred to this hospital from Malta in 1937.[38] The Gozo hospital closed down in December 1956 due to lack of patients.[39] The number of known lepers in the Maltese Islands in 1957 was 151 (a rate of 64 per 100,000 population).[40]

The decrease in the number of patients allowed for the eventual transfer of St Bartholomew Hospital to Hal Ferha Estate in Gharghur (an abandoned gun battery) in 1974. St Bartholomew Hospital was renamed Sptar Ruzar Briffa in 1973 to commemorate the physician who had been a torchbearer in the control of leprosy.[41] After its closure as a leprosarium, it was taken over to augment the geriatric services at St Vincent de Paule Residence.[42]

---

[36] Report on the Working of Government Departments during the financial years 1935-37. Government Printing Office, Malta, 1937-38, 2 vols., 1935-36:195; 1936-37:302
[37] *Report 1935-37*, op. cit.
[38] Bernard AV. *Annual Report on the Health Conditions of the Maltese Islands and on the work of the Medical and Health Department for the year 1937*. Government Printing Office, Malta, 1938, xlii.
[39] Farrer-Brown L, Boldero H, Oldham JB. *Report of the Medical Services Commission*. Central Office of Information, Malta, 1957, 24.
[40] Galea & Bonnici, 1957, *op. cit.*
[41] Cassar P. A torch-bearer in the control of leprosy in Malta. *Sunday Times [of Malta]*, 26 February 1995: 59
[42] *A Healthy People – A Happy People*. Ministry of Health, Malta, 1981, 10-11

Twenty-two residual cases were transferred to Hal Ferha Estate in December 1974. Each resident was provided with a self-contained flatlet having a sitting-bedroom, a kitchenette, and bathroom. They were further allotted land wherein to grow crops and carry out husbandry to generate income. Their medical needs were cared for by a nurse-on-duty and a doctor-on-call. They received six-monthly reviews by the leprologists. By 1987, only six residents (average age 67 years) remained. Some of these had been for almost fifty years in residential care. By 1994 only five residents – two females and three males – remained in the leprosarium. In 2001, the only remaining inmate was transferred to St. Vincent de Paule's geriatric hospital and Hal Ferha Estate was closed down.[43]

The previously treated cases of Hansen's Disease now live in the community. The head of households where these individuals live are entitled to receive a non-contributory Leprosy Pension from the Social Security Services.[44] These individuals are now generally elderly individuals whose numbers are slowing dwindling with a total of 32 individuals being reported in 2015 having decreased from the 43 cases registered in 2010. This suggests a current prevalence of treated victims of Hansen's disease of 7.2 per 100,000 population.[45] A new imported case of Hansen's Disease was identified in 2019. [46]

	2010	*2011*	*2012*	*2013*	*2014*	*2015*
expenditure	92,955	86,579	82,955	75,127	76,031	67,000
Beneficiaries - Male	29	28	24	23	23	
Beneficiaries - Female	14	14	12	10	11	
Beneficiaries - Total	43	42	36	33	34	32

Table 2: Statistics: Comparative Social Security Non-Contributory Benefits – Leprosy benefits
[Source: National Statistics Office]

The medical authorities in Malta have always been on the forefront in the treatment of leprosy. At the time of the Asylum's opening in 1900 until 1915, the crude Chaulmoogra oil constituted the only anti-leprosy treatment. This was poorly tolerated by the patients and treatment was often refused and ineffective. After 1918, a number of preparations were made available with varying success.[47] The development of antibiotics led to experiments with the use of these substances in the management of leprosy. By 1962, it was observed that multiple drug therapy could be efficacious. By 1962, it had become evident that the combined antibiotic therapy protocol was the most efficacious. In June 1972 a Leprosy eradication project was initiated in Malta

---

[43] Palmier BM. *Why did Hansen's Disease (Leprosy) in Malta persist until 2000 A.D*. Dissertation, Diploma in History of Medicine, Soc. Of Apothecaries, U.K., September 2003, +20p.
[44] *https://socialsecurity.gov.mt/en/Medical-Assistance/Pages/Leprosy-Assistance-.aspx*
[45] *Social Protection: Malta and the EU 2015*. Valletta: National Statistics Office, 2016, xviii, 84p.;   NSO News Release 053/2016, 29 March 2016
[46] W.H.O. Global Leprosy (Hansen disease) update, 2019: time to step-up prevention initiatives. *Weekly Epidemiological Report*. 4 September 2020; 36:417-440
[47] Galea & Bonnici, 1957, *op. cit*.

estimated to include about 300 patients. This project was jointly funded by the Sovereign Military Order of Malta (SMOM) in collaboration with the German Leprosy Association and the Malta Government. The project was eventually approved by the World Health Organization. The project was led by Professor Enno Freerksen, Director of the Borstel Research Institute of Hamburg. Two Maltese physicians – Dr. George Depasquale and Dr Edgar Bonnici – were enrolled in the project, aided by Dr Anton Agius Ferrante.[48] The new treatment regimen chosen was based on the Freerksen's trial which combined treatment with rifampicin, isoniazid (INH), prothionamide, and diaminodiphenylsulfone (DDS). The Malta Project was concluded formally in December 1999, and there have been no case of endemic leprosy reported since.[49] The Multiple Drug Therapy regimen as pioneered in Malta, however using instead a combination of dapsone, rifampicin, and clofazimine, is still the best treatment for preventing nerve damage, deformity, disability, and further transmission. Leprosy is now considered "extinct" on the Maltese Islands with no cases being reported in the Maltese native population. However, vigilance is still required in the light of the present problem of irregular immigration from the African coast from regions where the disease is still prevalent.

---

[48] Buttigieg & Micallef Stafrace, 2008, *op. cit.*
[49] Freerksen E, Rosenfeld M, Depasquale G, Bonnici E, Gatt P. The Malta Project--a country freed itself of leprosy. A 27-year progress study (1972-1999) of the first successful eradication of leprosy. *Chemotherapy*. 2001; 47:309-331

Biography: Prominent Maltese leprologists

The Hospital for Lepers sited in the Poor House was established in 1900. The day-to-day medical care of the inmates was generally furnished by the resident medical staff – the Resident Superintendent and Assistant Resident Superintendent – responsible for the Hospital for Incurables forming part of the poor House Complex. These, during the period 1900-1938, included:

Alfredo Marras MD.

Education: University of Malta qualified M.D. 1883.
Career: Appointed as Resident Superintendent for the Hospital for Incurables in April 1895. He retained his post until 1902 when he was appointed Resident Medical Superintendent to the Central Hospital in Malta.

Ermanno E. Micallef MD.

Education: University of Malta qualified M.D. 1895.
Career: Appointed as Assistant Resident Superintendent for the Hospital for Incurables in September 1898 assuming the post of Resident Superintendent in December 1902. He retained his post until 1932.

Salvatore Portelli MD

Education: University of Malta qualified M.D. 1898.
Career: Appointed as Assistant Resident Superintendent for the Hospital for Incurables in December 1902. He retained his post until 1916.

Marco Samuele Marguerat MD

Education: University of Malta qualified M.D. 1892.
Career: First appointed with the Health Department as a District Medical Officer for Siggiewi, Malta since June 1902. Appointed as Assistant Resident Superintendent for the Hospital for Incurables in January 1917. He retained his post until 1929.

William Aquilina MD

Education: University of Malta qualified M.D. 1916.
Career: First appointed with the Health Department as a District Medical Officer for Tarxien – Paola – Gudia – Luqa district, Malta since July 1920. Appointed as Junior Assistant Resident Superintendent for the Hospital for Incurables in July 1928, Assistant Resident Superintendent in May 1929, and Resident Superintendent in 1941. He retained his post until 1934.

Salvatore Muscat
MD
b. 1880; d. 1962

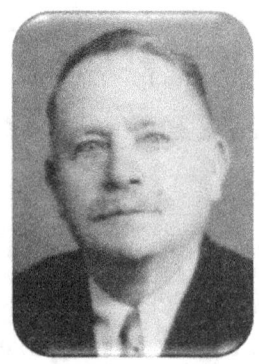

Education: University of Malta qualified M.D. 1907.

Career: First appointed with the Health Department as Resident Assistant in April 1909, later Superintendent at Connaught Hospital after January 1917. Appointed as Assistant Resident Superintendent for the Hospital for Incurables in October 1932 and eventually Resident Superintendent until his retirement in 1941.

Joseph Bugeja
MD

Education: University of Malta qualified M.D. 1925. In 1930, attended an 8-week course at the School of Tropical Medicine – Calcutta and visited several leprosy hospitals in India.

Career: First appointed with the Health Department serving as Assistant Medical Officer at the Malta Central Hospital since October 1927. Appointed as Junior Assistant Resident Superintendent for the Hospital for Incurables in May 1929, Assistant Resident Superintendent in December 1934 retired 1941. *Achievements:* He presented a very detailed report about the state of Hansen Disease in Malta up to 1929.

Bibliography: J. Bugeja: Leprosy in Malta. Reports on the working of Government departments during the financial year 1930-31. Government Printing Office, Malta, 1932, R:p.17-30

John G. Cutajar Beck
MD

Education: University of Malta qualified M.D. 1922.

Career: First appointed with the Health Department serving as Superintendent at Connaught Hospital, Malta since January 1917. Appointed as Junior Resident Medical Officer for the Hospital for Incurables in July 1929; Assistant Resident Superintendent in December 1934 and Resident Superintendent in December 1941.

Dr. Edgar Dandria
MD

Education: University of Malta qualified M.D. 1928.

Career: First appointed with the Health Department serving as Assistant Medical Officer to Santo Spirito Hospital since July 1933. Appointed as Junior Resident Medical Officer for the Hospital for Incurables in December 1934; retired 1941 on abolition of post.

Bibliography: Malta Blue Books – 1821-1938. https://nso.gov.mt/Home/ABOUT_NSO/Historical_Statistics/Malta_Blue_Books/Pages/Malta-Blue-Book-1938.aspx

Dr. Richard Toledo MD	*Education:* University of Malta qualified M.D. 1934. *Career:* Medical Superintendent for St. Bartholomew Hospital, retired 1940. After his retirement, remained active philanthropically to raise funds to support entertainment projects in the hospital.
Dr. Edgar Bonnici MD	*Career:* Medical Superintendent for St. Bartholomew Hospital. *Achievements:* During his tenure, treatment for Hansen Disease with antibiotics was experimented with. In 1947, he observed on the effect of streptomycin and concluded that "perhaps combined treatment with streptomycin and sulphones (Diasone) might prove of greater therapeutic value."

Department of Health: Annual Reports on the Health Conditions of the Maltese Islands and on the work of the Medical and Health Department for the years 1937-1971. Department of Health, Malta, 1938-1972, annual reports

Individuals who further contributed to the care and welfare of the victims of Hansen Disease were the medical professionals who were appointed to the post of Medical Officers in charge of the Venereal & Dermatology Department.

Vincent M. Curmi MD

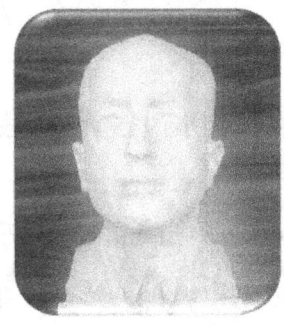

Education: University of Naples qualified M.D. ~1920 [undetermined but sometime between 1915-1925].

Career: First appointed with the Health Department as a medical inspector of the Sanitary Branch under the terms of Ordinance VI of 1920 in April 1925. Appointed Medical Officer in charge of the Venereal & Dermatology Department at the Civil Hospital in Floriana, Malta in November 1926. He continued in the latter post until his retirement in January 1951. His appointment allowed him to continue to serve the general public in private practice as well. He was appointed lecturer in Venerology & Dermatology at the University of Malta in January 1930, a post he held until his retirement as professor in 1951. *Achievements:* His period leading the venerology & dermatology department was marked by the introduction of antibiotics in the pharmaceutical armamentarium - presenting an opportunity for Dr Curmi to experiment with the use of these medications in the management of venereal disease [syphilis, gonorrhoea, etc.] - he describes his observations with the use of these medication in the annual reports presented and published by the Department of Health. He was also required to face the increased prevalence of skin disorders [e.g., scabies] during the war years.

Bibliography: Malta Blue Books – 1821-1938.
https://nso.gov.mt/Home/ABOUT_NSO/Historical_Statistics/Malta_Blue_Books/Pages/Malta-Blue-Book-1938.aspx

Rosario Briffa
BSc, BPharm, MD
b. 1906, d.1963

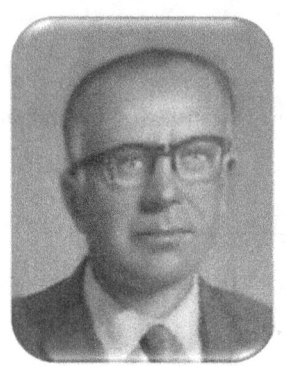

Education: Malta Lyceum, University of Malta qualified B.Sc. (1928), B.Pharm. (1928), and M.D. (1931); awarded scholarships to follow postgraduate courses in dermatology and tropical disease at the Institute of Dermatology and St Thomas Hospital in London and the Calcutta School of Tropical Disease. *Career:* First appointed Junior Assistant Medical Officer at the Central Hospital in October 1932 being seconded to the dermatology department. In March 1938, appointed Leprosy Control Officer and eventually Assistant Medical Officer to the Venerology and Dermatology Department. In 1944, appointed Visiting Physician to St Bartholomew Leper Hospital, and in January 1951 appointed senior consultant in skin disease at the Central Hospital and Chambray Hospital; also nominated honorary skin disease specialist at the Malta War Memorial Hospital for Children. In 1950, appointed to the post of lecturer on dermatology and venerology at the University of Malta. *Achievements:* His work as Leprosy Control Officer was marked by the introduction of a number of significant changes in the medical and social management of leprosy. He was also one of the literary giants in the field of Maltese literature and co-founder of the *Ghaqda tal-Malti* in 1931.

Bibliography: C. Briffa: Briffa, Ruzar. In: M.J. Sciavone, L.J. Scerri (eds.): *Maltese Biographies of the twentieth century*. PIN, Malta, 1997, p.93-94; P. Cassar: A torch-bearer in the control of leprosy. *Sunday Times (Malta)*, 26th February 1995, p.59

Anthony Agius Ferrante
MD, PHC

Education: University of Malta qualified M.D. (1946), PHC. In 1955, attended course of training in Dermatology in the United Kingdom and visited a number of hospitals on the continent. *Career:* Joined the 1st King's Own Malta Regiment Surgeon-Captain in August 1954 and eventually commissioned as Temporary Surgeon-Captain in the Royal Malta Artillery in May 1959 retaining the post until September 1965. *Achievements:* His tenure was marked by the initiation of the Leprosy Eradication Project of Malta that led to the eradication of Hansen Disease from the Islands.

Bibliography: Surgeon-Captain Anthony Agius Ferrante MD PHC. Medical Officers of the Malta Garrison. https://www.maltaramc.com/regsurg/a/agiusferrante.html [information from *The Army List March 1965*, London HM Stationery Office 1965].

The Leprosy Eradication Project of Malta that led to the eradication of Hansen Disease from the Islands was managed by Drs. George Depasquale MD (Melit. 1969), Edgar Bonnici MD, Cecil Tancred Paris MD (Melit. 1958), and William Grima MD (Melit. 1940). The project was subsequently followed up by Dr. Paul Gatt MD (Melit. 1984) FRCPEd.

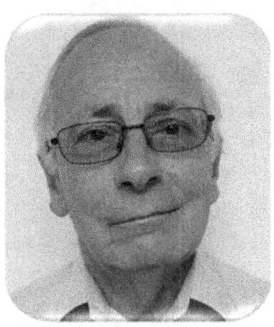

George Depasquale
MD [Melit] 1969
Served as principal leprologist 1972-1989

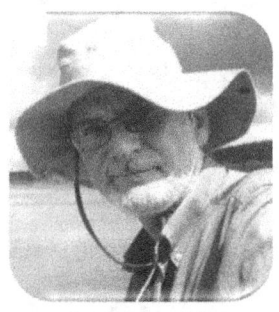

Paul Gatt
MD [Melit] 1984, FRCP(Edin)
Served as principal leprologist 1990-2004

Bibliography: A. Agius-Ferrante, G. Depasquale, E. Bonnici, C. Paris, W. Grima: The leprosy eradication-project of Malta. *Z Tropenmed Parasitol.*, 1973, 24:Suppl 1:p.49-52; E. Freerksen, M. Rosenfeld, G. Depasquale, E. Bonnici, P. Gatt: The Malta Project--a country freed itself of leprosy. A 27-year progress study (1972-1999) of the first successful eradication of leprosy. *Chemotherapy*, 2001, 47(5):p.309-331

Maltese Leprosaria

Reports on the various leprosaria with patient population and financial costs can be found in the annual reports published by the Office of Charitable Institutions [1900-1936] and the Department of Health [1936-1971].

Hospitalis Sanctj Franciscj, Malta

This hospital, sited just outside the wall of the Medieval capital Mdina in Malta, is documented to have been functioning by 1372, though its establishment date was earlier possibly around 1299. On the 20th July – 7th August 1299, Pope Boniface VIII appoints Cardinal Bishop Gerardus of Sabina as an Apostolic Legate to the Kingdom of Sicily [including Malta] who is authorised to grant up to a hundred days of indulgence to the faithful who assist in the building of churches and the running of hospitals.[1] The hospital was managed by members of the Franciscan Order who included the care of lepers in their vocation. It has been suggested by Dr. Gerlach [as reported by Dr. Giovanni Gulia] that on the basis of its locality outside the walls of the city and the Franciscan Order management, the establishment had been initially set up to serve as a leprosarium. No documentary proof has however been found to substantiate this assertion.[2] The hospital became known as Santo Spirito Hospital in 1467. By 1494, the hospital documentation makes no mention of lepers but refers only to "*poveri abitanti*".[3]

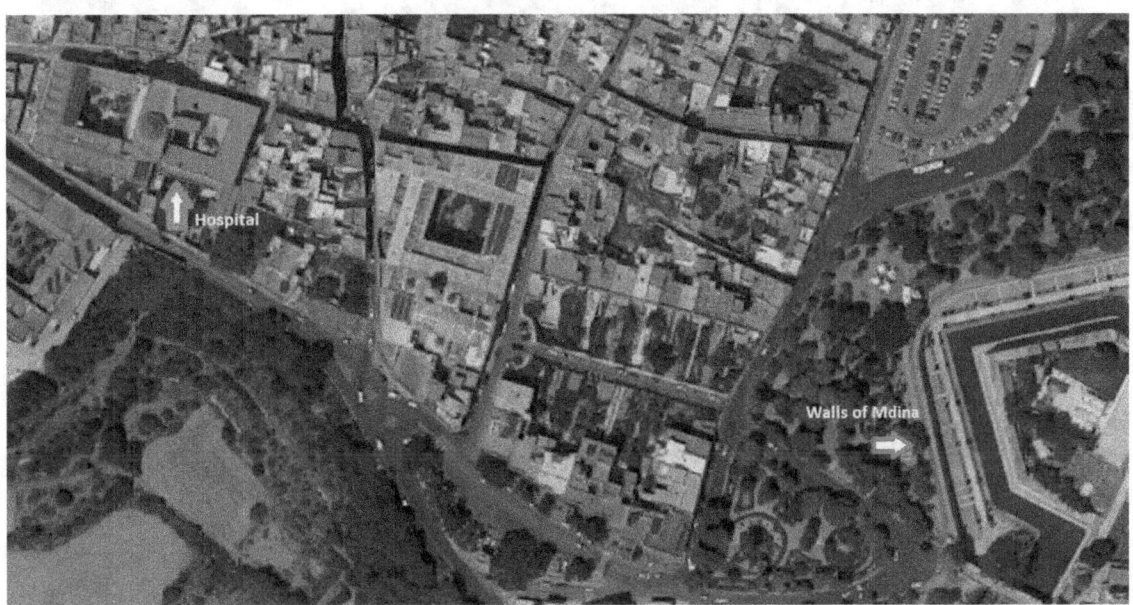

1. *Reg. Vat. F f.ccxlviiiii-ccliii verso, ep.xxiii*. Transcribed in: Aquilina GA, Fiorini S, editors. *Documentary Sources of Maltese history. Part IV Documents at the Vatican. No. 2 Archivio Segreto Vaticano: Cancellaria Apostolica and Camera Apostolica and related sources at the Biblioteca Apostolica Vaticana 416-1479*. University Press, Malta, 2005, doc.41, ep. XXIII, 63-64.
2. Gulia G. Sopra un caso de Lebbra dei Greci. *Il Barth*, 29 January 1874, 3(19):372-377.
3. Fiorini S. *Santo Spirito Hospital at Rabat, Malta – The early years to 1575*. Department of information, Malta, 1989.

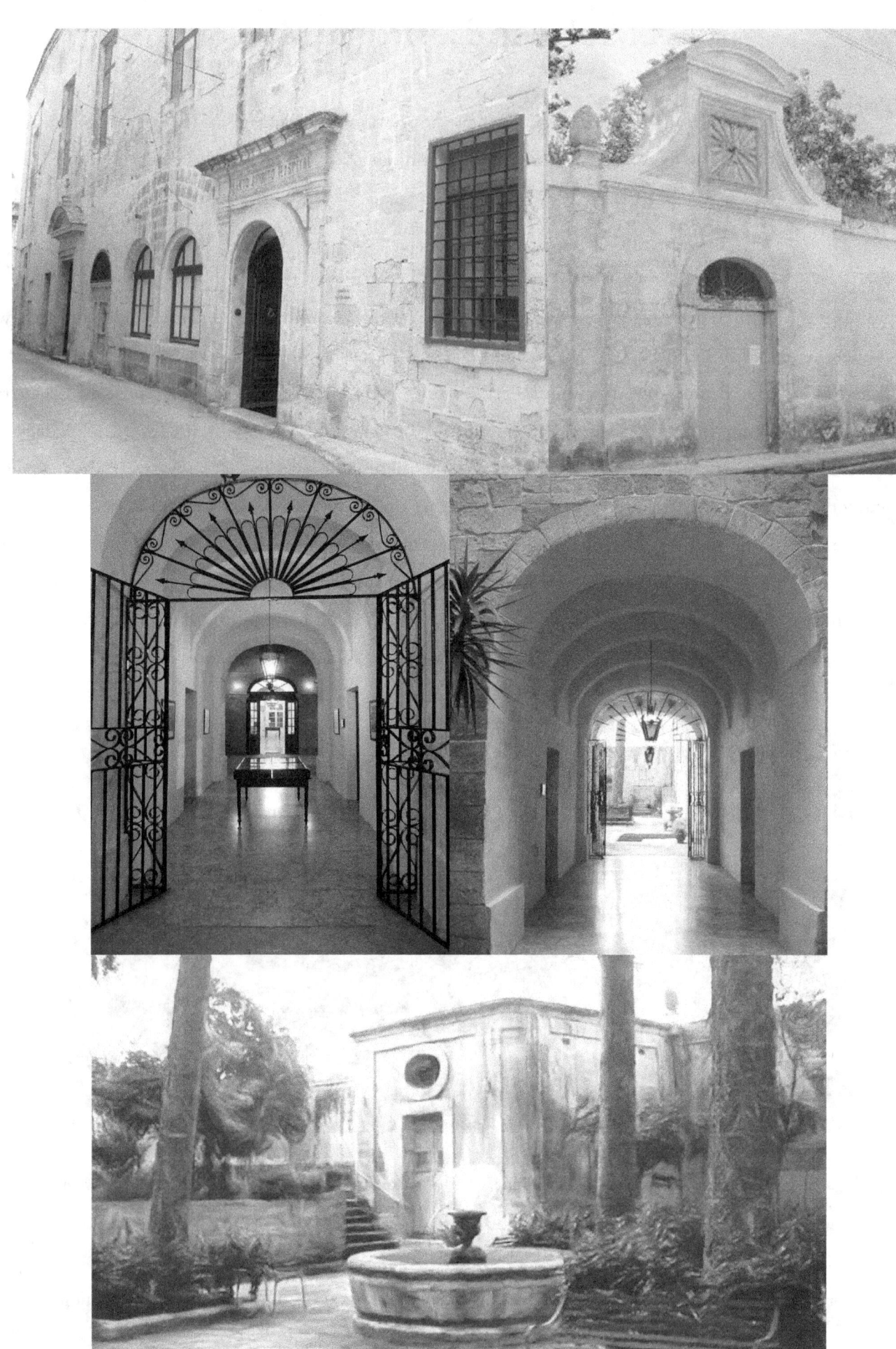

Hospitalis Sanctj Franciscj, Malta [modern views]

St. Bartholomew Hospital, Malta

Established as a separate building in the "Poor House - St. Vincent de Paule Hospital" grounds in 1900. Originally occupied by males only; female wing opened in 1912. The hospital population reached its high-water mark in 1917 with 114 inmates (71 males; 43 females). The leprosarium was named St. Bartholomew Hospital in 1937. In 1956, the leprosarium was described as an old but fine and spacious building with a bed complement of 118 beds. However during 1953-54, it only housed an average of 74 patients. The hospital had better amenities than many of the other hospitals in Malta. The wards, corridors and gardens were noted to be spacious and pleasing. There was an entertainment hall and efforts were being made to organize shows and outings for the inmates. The hospital was managed by one medical officer, the Medical Superintendent, who was relieved by one of the doctors at contiguous St Vincent de Paule Hospital on his off-days. The building was renamed Ruzar Briffa Hospital in 1973 to commemorate the physician who had been a torch-bearer in the control of leprosy. The decrease in the number of patients following the Leprosy Eradication Project of 1972 allowed for the closure of St Bartholomew Hospital in the late 1970s and in February 1980 was taken over to augment the geriatric services at St Vincent de Paule Hospital (now renamed Has-Serh Hospital).

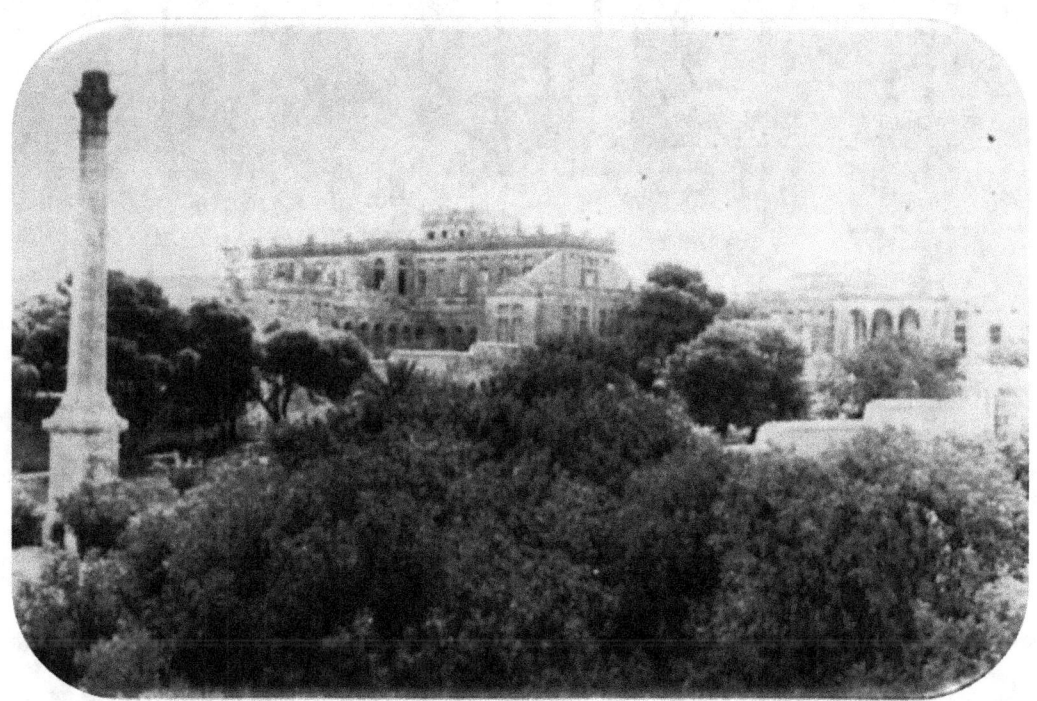

1. Office of Charitable Institutions: *Reports on the Workings of Government Departments during the financial years 1900-1936*. Government Printing Office, Malta, 1901-1937, annual reports.
2. Department of Health: *Annual Reports on the Health Conditions of the Maltese Islands and on the work of the Medical and Health Department for the years 1937-1971*. Department of Health, Malta, 1938-1972, annual reports.
3. L. Farrer-Brown, H. Boldero, J.B. Oldham: *Report of the Medical Services Commission*. Central Office of Information, Malta, 1957, p.24.

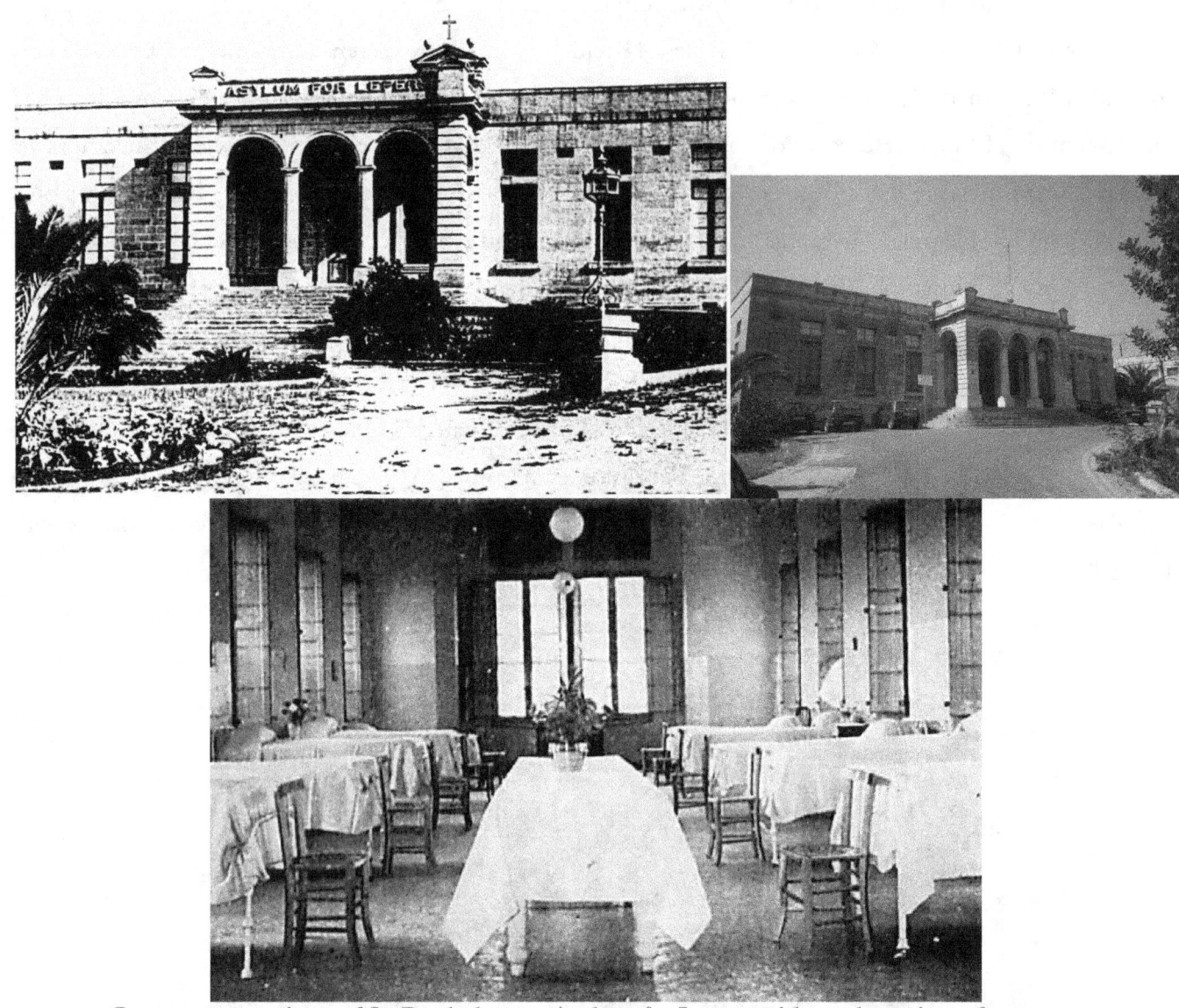
Contemporary views of St. Bartholomew Asylum for Lepers with modern view of entrance

Sacred Heart Hospital, Gozo

Established in 1937 in the building previously used as the Married Quarters at Fort Chambray in Gozo. The Sacred Heart Hospital in Gozo, had a bed complement of 27 beds. Thirteen men and two women, originally from Gozo, were transferred to this hospital from Malta in 1937. The patients were cared for by two sisters of Charity, one of whom served as Matron, two male and two female nurses. The spiritual needs were catered for by a Chaplain. The medical needs were catered for by the two physicians assigned to Victoria Hospital at Victoria-Rabat in Gozo. The Gozo hospital closed down in December 1956 due to lack of patients.

1. Department of Health: *Annual Reports on the Health Conditions of the Maltese Islands and on the work of the Medical and Health Department for the years 1937-1971*. Department of Health, Malta, 1938-1972, annual reports.
2. L. Farrer-Brown, H. Boldero, J.B. Oldham: *Report of the Medical Services Commission*. Central Office of Information, Malta, 1957, p.24.

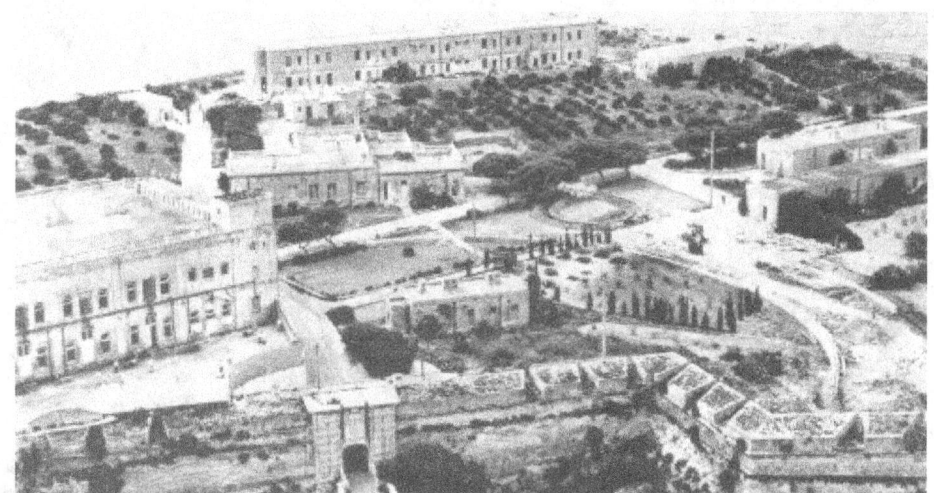

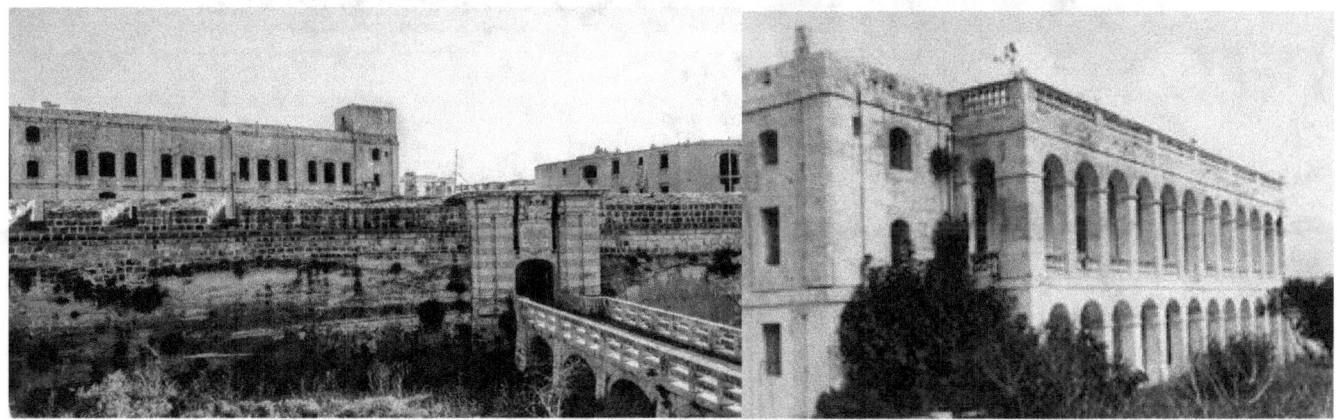

Sacred Heart Hospital, Gozo

Hal Ferha Estate, Malta

In 1974, the closure of St Bartholomew's Leprosarium at the Mgieret Hospice to be used as an extension of the Hospice for the Elderly, brought up the need to provide alternative accommodation for the remaining treated but institutionalised victims of Hansen's disease [leprosy] that then numbered 22 individuals. The Gharghur Battery was transformed into an isolated residence with the construction of additional structures and including the provision of a nearby plot of land for the inmates to cultivate. The edifice became known as the Tal-Ferha Leprosarium. In 1989, there were only a few spent-out individuals apart from three active cases notified to the Medical and Health Department. By 1994, only five residents remained; by 2001 the last inmate was transferred to the state geriatric's hospital. The Tal-Ferha Leprosarium formally closed in 2004 and was left completely abandoned.

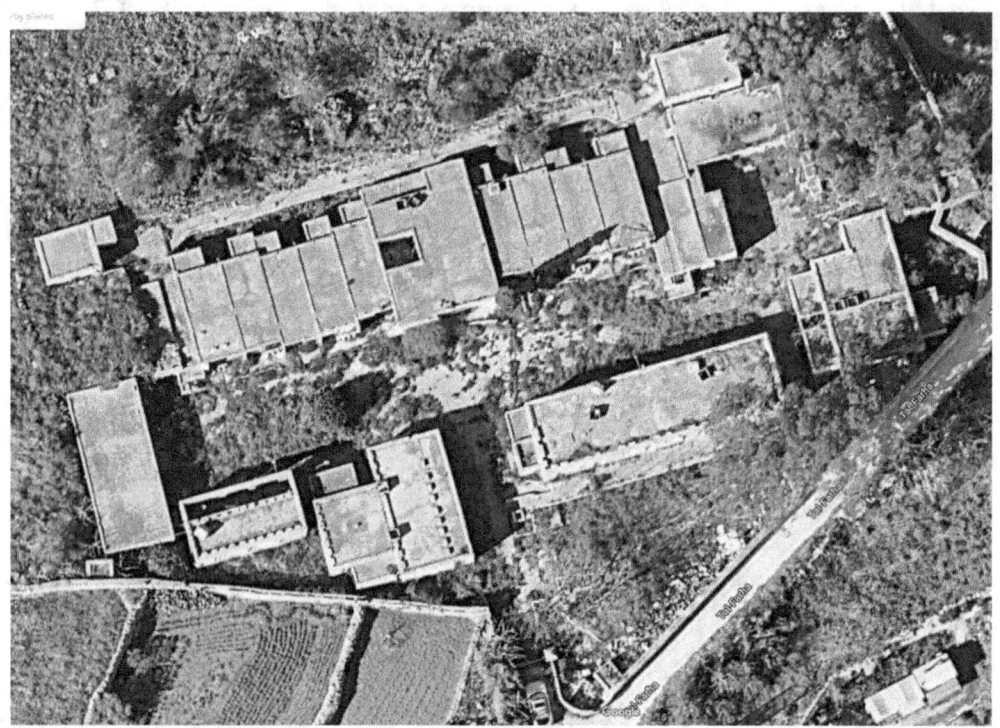

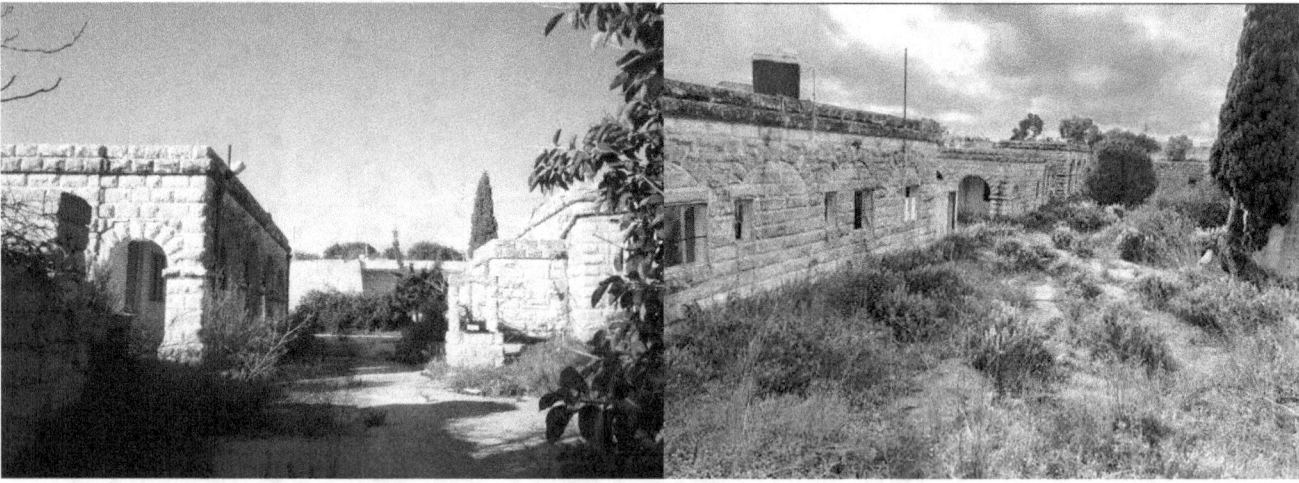

Present day views of Hal Ferha Leprosarium, Malta

Support Organizations in Malta

Military & Hospitaller Order of St. Lazarus of Jerusalem

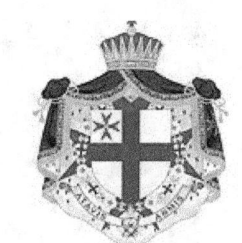

The Order of St. Lazarus was originally instituted as a hospitaller Order in Jerusalem after 1090 with the specific purpose of caring for sufferers of leprosy. The presence of the Order of St Lazarus in Malta was a relatively late occurrence. The Order of St. Lazarus in the Maltese owes its presence in the Maltese Islands to the traditional Anglo-Maltese links established during the nineteenth and twentieth century and dates only to the latter third of the twentieth century. In the mid-1960s, a number of Maltese individuals were admitted to the International Order. The Maltese members of the Order, in 1966, established their own *Independent Commandery of Malta* with the aim of helping 'by medical and non-medical means in the prevention and management of chronic long-drawn disease in the population of these Islands, and to minimize the consequences thereof'. This commandery, in April 1969, was raised to the status of a priory with the title of "Priory of Malta". The Roll of Member of the Order published in 1969 includes 17 Maltese members among a list of 500 members worldwide. The Priory of Malta continued to increase its membership. It was elevated to its present status of Grand Priory of the Maltese Islands after the Order established its Chancery in Malta in 1973. By 1983, the Grand Priory of Malta was represented by 55 members. In 2005, the Maltese jurisdiction expanded its services in Gozo by the establishment of the Commandery of Gozo. Another branch of the Military & Hospitaller Order of St. Lazarus of Jerusalem in Malta was established in 1973, known as initially as the *Hereditary Commandery of Lochore in Malta*, to cater for British residents. After 2004, the jurisdiction started admitting Maltese members to supplement the dwindling British membership. This was renamed the Commandery of the Castello in 1986 and Grand Commandery in 2009.

The Grand Priory of the Maltese Islands has maintained an active philanthropic target to collected funds to assist the amelioration of the social conditions of sufferers of Hansen's disease in countries where the disease remains particularly rife, such as Kenya and Egypt. It also contributes to other worthy charitable causes not linked to leprosy. In 1994, it set up a dedicated Leprosy Fund amounting to an overall value of Lm3,000 [~€7,000] with the aim of distributing the funds over a three-year period to Caritas-Egypt to assist in the treatment of lepers at the Abu-Zabaal Leprosy Mission that consisted of a mud-brick "leprosy village" of some 200 families. Inhabitants there were given medical assistance and training in crafts. In the subsequent five years further donations amounting to about Lm2,400 [~€5,600] were collected to support the establishment of the St. Lazarus Leprosy Mission in Pumwani, Kenya managed by Fr. Publius Cassar, and to assist lepers in Ethiopia and Madras. Since very early on in its existence, the Grand Priory also undertook to organize social activities for the institutionalized leper community in Malta. In 1971, it provided a television set to serve the needs if the female inmates of St. Bartholomew Hospital.

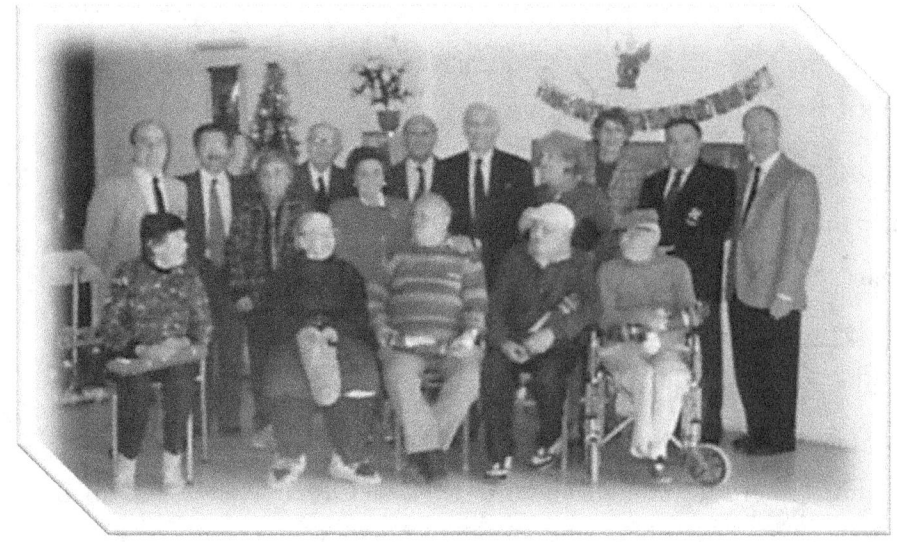

Christmas Party at Hal Ferha Leprosarium, December 1995

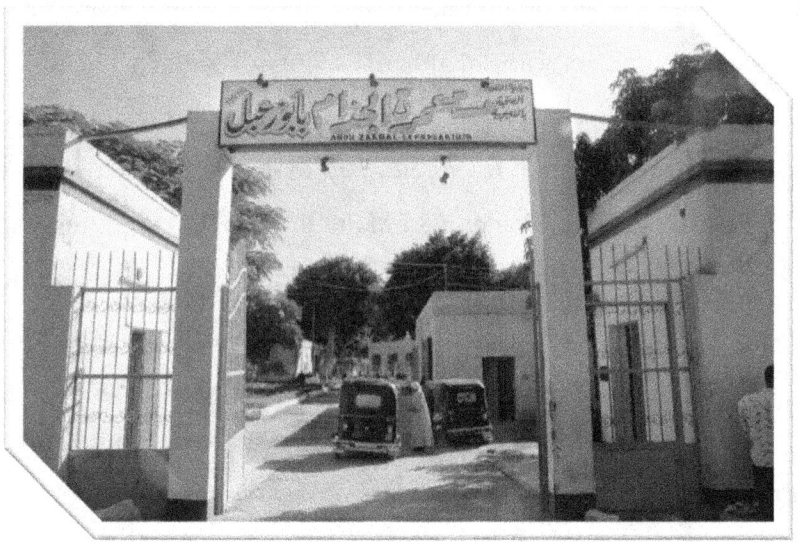

Caritas-Egypt Abu-Zabaal Leprosy Mission

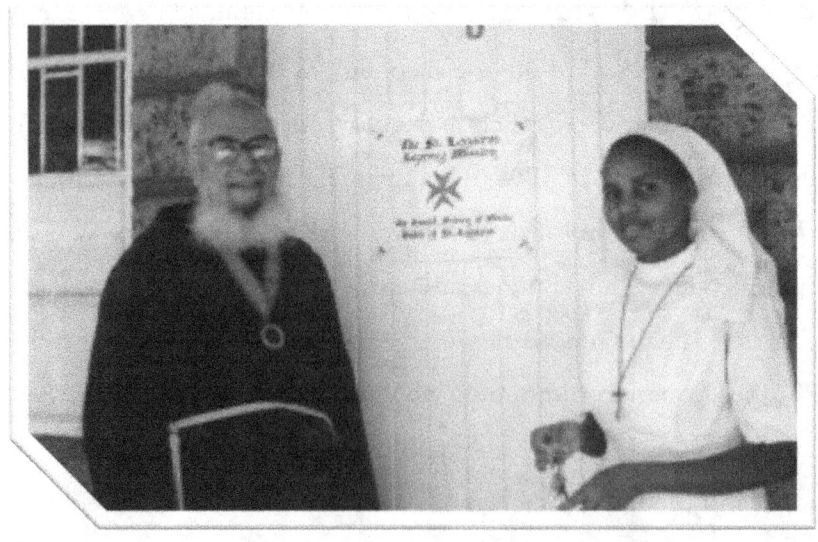

Fr. Publius Cassar at the St. Lazarus Leprosy Mission, in Kenya, 1996

The activities of the Grand Priory in favour of the fight against leprosy persisted even after the closure of the last institution housing victims of Hansen Disease. Activities were organized to specifically support the work being done by Maltese missionary workers with victims of Hansen Disease overseas. The receiving organizations included the Missionary Movement "Gesu fil-Proxmu" managed by Fr. George Grima with donations being made to build a school for children affected by leprosy in Ethiopia in 2007, and to the Working hands project that is a UK Registered Charity managed by hand surgeon Dr. Donald Sammut running a surgical programme, based at a leprosy hospital in Nepal, supporting a team of Hand Surgeons who travel there to operate and to teach the local surgeons.

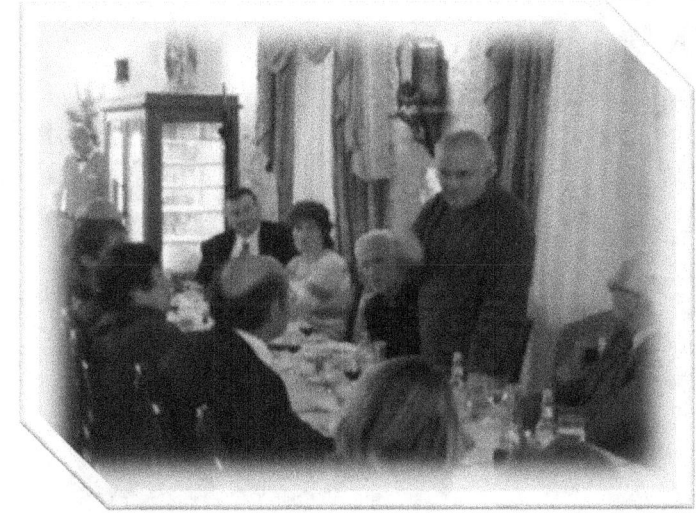
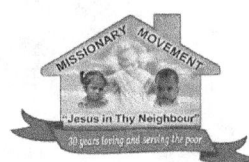

Presentation to Fr. G. Grima to support work with lepers in Ethiopia - 16th December 2007

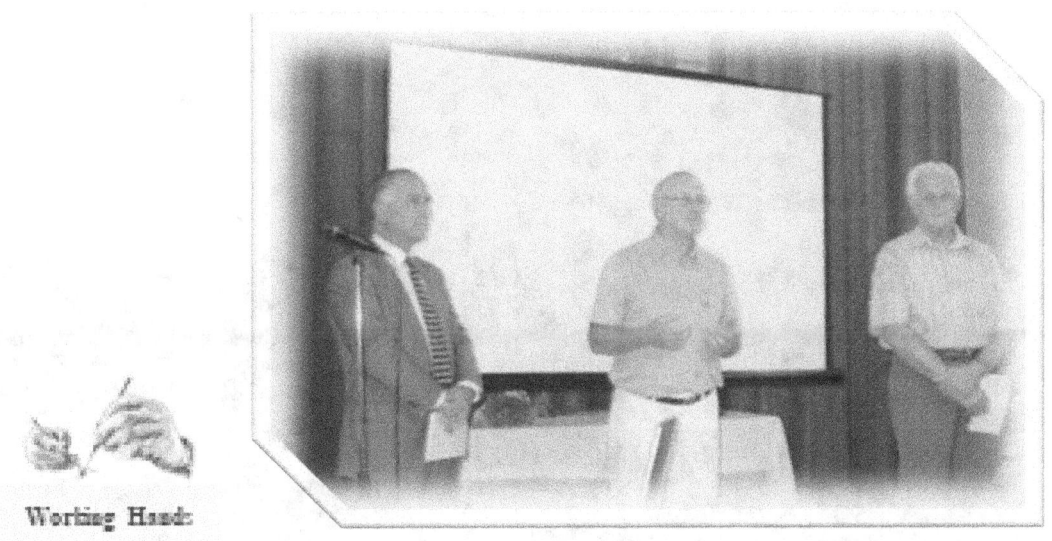

Presentation to Dr. Donald Sammut representing Working Hands - 12th September 2008

The Grand Priory further supported the LEPRA Foundation (The British Leprosy Relief Association) by assisting in fund-raising enterprises to help support measures aimed at eradicating the disease and the Artificial Hands Project. It also organized annual meetings with public lectures delivered on World Leprosy Day and to use the public media through articles and talk-shows aimed at increasing the awareness of the suffering experienced by the victims of this physically and socially destructive disease. It also collaborated with the Oxford-based International Leprosy Association's Global Project on the *History of Leprosy* funded by the Nippon Foundation providing relevant documentation about the disease in Malta. It further provided support to a research initiative aiming to determine the genetic predisposition to becoming infected with *Mycobacterium*. In 2009, it was asked to assume the responsibility of an existing voluntary organization – the Raoul Follereau Foundation [Malta] : Order of Charity – whose aim was to collect funds to support the fight against Hansen Disease.

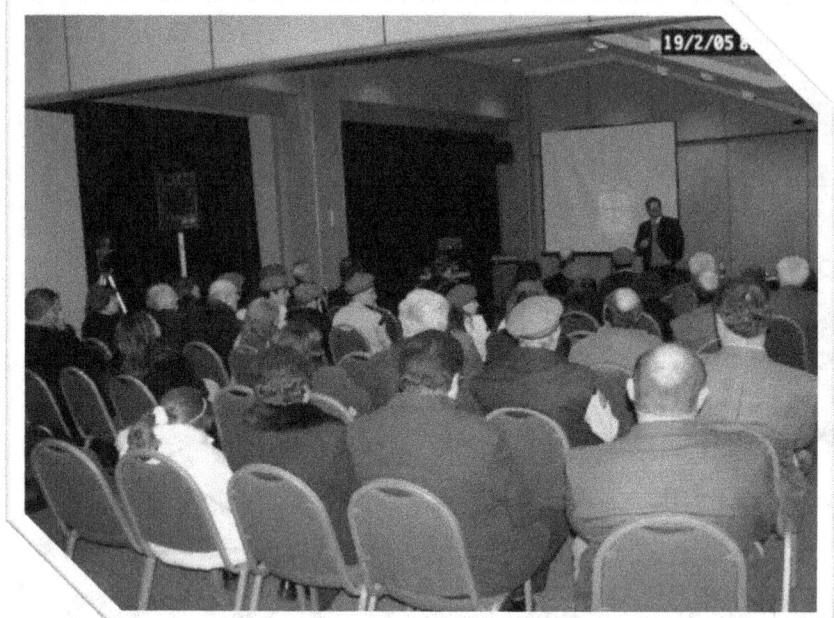
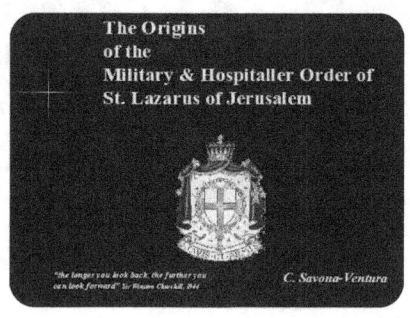
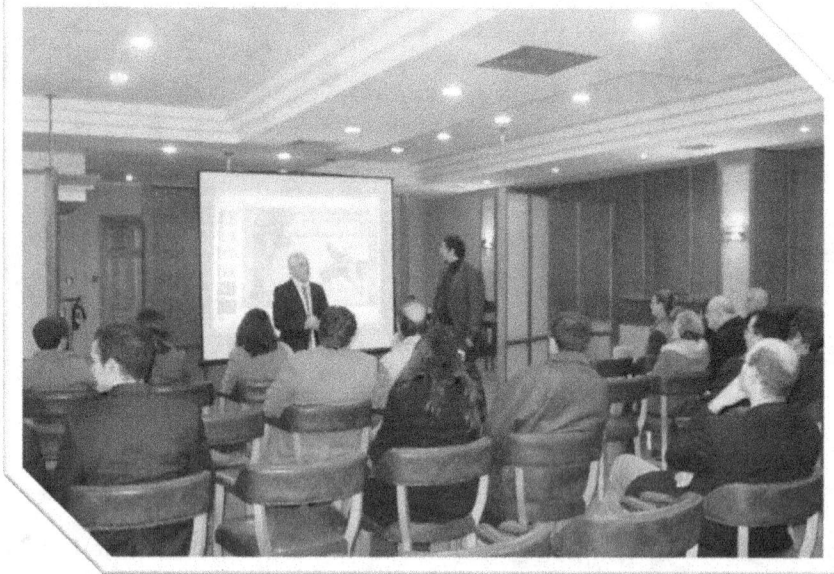
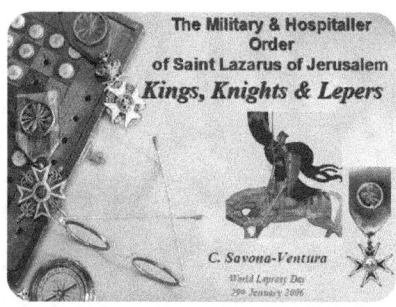

Annual lectures delivered on World Leprosy Day

The Grand Commandery of the Castello has in the last decade maintained an active philanthropic activity to assist the amelioration of the social conditions of sufferers of Hansen's disease in countries where the disease remains particularly rife. It also contributes to other worthy charitable causes not linked to leprosy. Leprosy-related projects sponsored by the Grand commandery included support for the Leper colony in the Sichaun Province of China named the Jing Yang Village. Work consisted of building a health clinic and providing water to all the dwellings in the village. The agreement was 'that should we be in a position to raise all the required sum of £25,000 Sterling within a certain period of time, we would be allowed to fly the flag of St Lazarus on top of the clinic'. The targeted sum was collected in just over 12 months. In addition, the jurisdiction supported a leper colony in Kazakhstan with a donation of €10,000 to enable badly-needed refurbishment of the bathrooms and to buy new beds; while in addition the Grand Commandery provided the Leah Pattison's Dattapur Leprosy centre in India with a much-needed ambulance and helped set up a hospice designed to treat chronically ill patients, especially those suffering from Hansen disease.

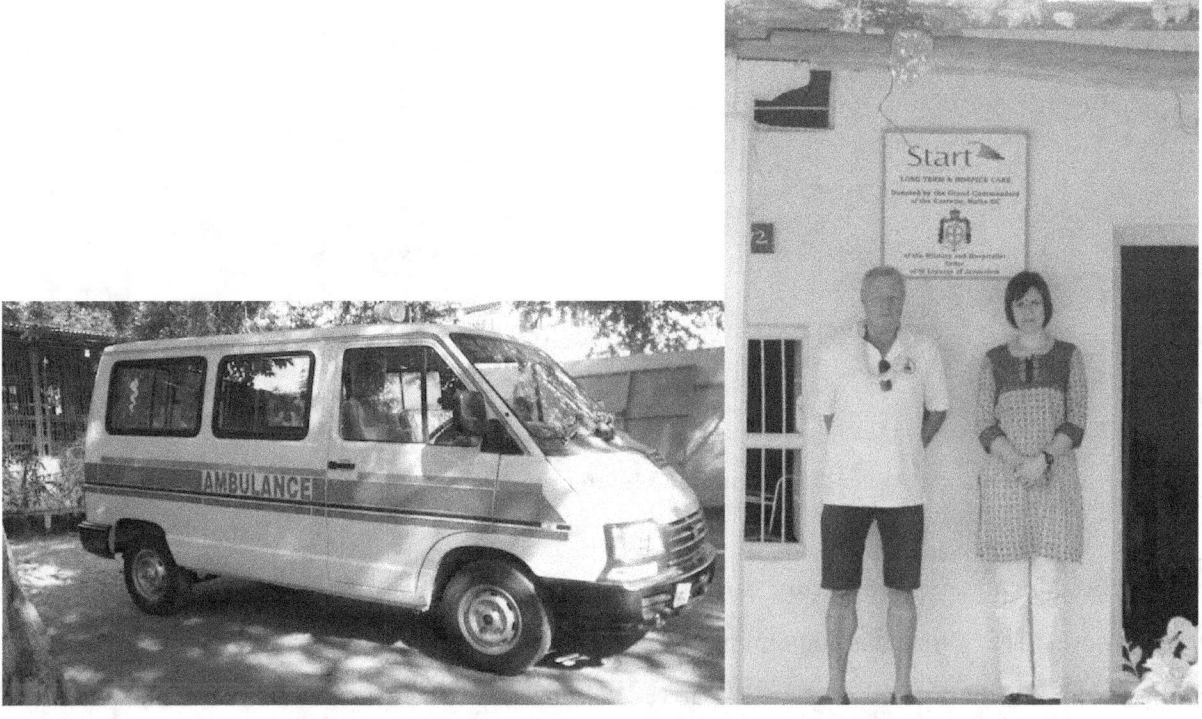

Donations to the Leah Pattison's Dattapur Leprosy centre in India

Raoul Follereau Foundation [Malta] – Order of Charity

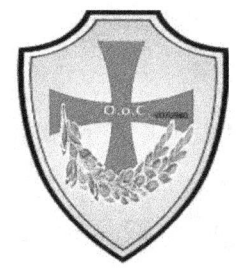

This voluntary organization was established in Malta in 1969 after signing an agreement with the International Raoul Follereau Foundation (est. 1946) with the aim of helping in the fight against leprosy in Malta and overseas. The aims of the organization are to encourage social help to those suffering from leprosy; to ascertain that these people are treated as they should; to help lepers find their place in society; and to give financial help to leprosaria and missions working with them. Funds to achieve these aims were regularly collected by a membership fee from the members subscribing to the organization and through donations. It maintained contact with the membership base through an annual newsletter. The organization also maintained regular contact with the Malta Leprosarium inmates providing hamper gifts and other items. It also organized memorial masses for Order of Charity members who died.

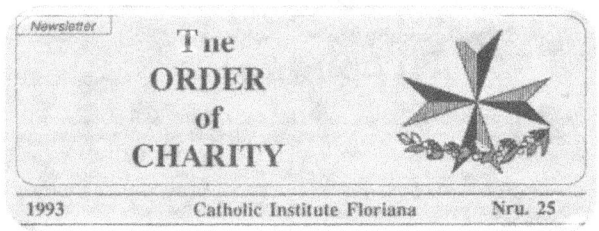

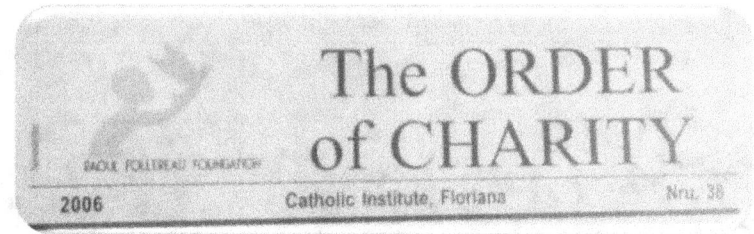

Newsletter Headers

The main bulk of the donations was made towards international organizations involved in the battle against Hansen's Disease, particularly those missions managed by Maltese missionaries. During the first 40 years of its existence, the Order of Charity had sent a total of Lm141,663 [equivalent to about €330,000]. In 1991, the sum of Lm4,157 (equivalent to about €9,700) was made to 25 recipients including:

Leprosy Control Program [Sierra Leone]	Sr. Anne Catania [Philippines]	Dr. Jose V. Fernando [Philippines]
CIOMAL (Culion)	Fr. Carm Attard SDB [India]	Fr. J. Damascene [India]
Medical Missionaries of Mary	Fr. Albert Said SJ [India]	Fr. Elias Menuba [Nigeria]
Damien Foundation	Fr. Publius Cassar OFM [Kenya]	Fr. Willy Tangi [Tanzania]
St. Francis Leprosy Guild	Fr. Nicholas Batipola [Sri Lanka]	Spigolatrice della Chiesa
German Leprosy Relief Assoc.	Fr. Dominic Buffour [Ghana]	G. Kapuluta [Tanzania]
Int. Fed. Anti-Leprosy Assoc.	Union Inter. Fond. Follereau	Sr. Kevin Hanley
Emmaus – Swiss	Assoc. Française Fond. Follereau	
Leprosy Mission	Amici de Raoul Follereau	

In 2009, the managing president George Spiteri approached the Grand Priory of the Maltese Islands – MHOSLJ to assume responsibility for the management of the Order of Charity. Statutory changes made to amalgamate the two organizations with the Raoul Follereau Foundation [Malta] – Order of Charity becoming thus a voluntary organization affiliate of the Grand Priory registered formally with the Malta Commissioner for Voluntary Organizations [V/O 0980]. The amount of donations were markedly augmented during 2014-2018 after the organization participated in the Weekend Mission Marathons using the media to collect donations for missionary projects. A decision was made to reduce the number of recipients in order that the donations made become of a significant value. In 2016, the recipient organizations included:

- Lepra U.K. Artificial Hands Project
- Capuchin Fathers
- Conventual Franciscan Fathers
- Sr. Ann Catanja [Philippine Mission]
- Sr. Maria Consage [Nigeria Mission]
- Prof. Horatio Vella [Ethiopian Mission]
- CIOMAL (Switzerland)
- Associatione Italiana Amici Raoul Follereau
- Damien Dutton Foundation, Belgium
- Association Française Raoul Follereau
- Direct monetary support to local lepers living in the community

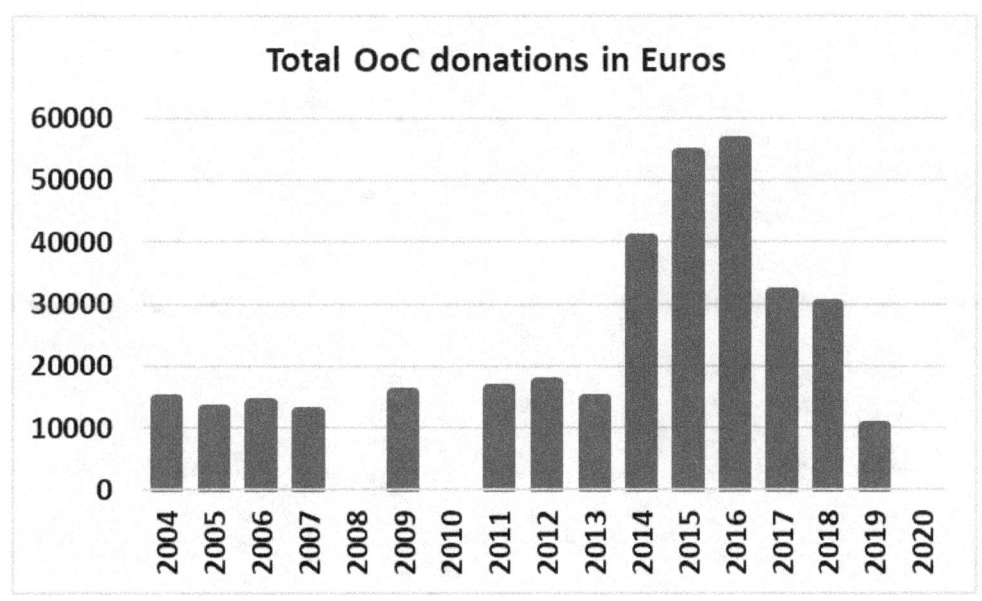

The Maltese Association of the Sovereign Military Order of Malta [SMOM-Malta]

The Malta branch of the Sovereign Military Order of Malta, originally the Order of St. John of Jerusalem, Rhodes and Malta, was established in Malta in 1960 with the first investiture ceremony in Malta being held 1967. As a local association, it set out to support a number of social initiatives. In respect to support towards the fight against Hansen Disease, the association was on the forefront is supporting the Malta Leprosy Project. This first leprosy eradication program involving widespread use of combination therapy started in Malta in June 1972. It was based on extensive experimental and clinical studies and was formally concluded on 31 December 1999. This project was jointly funded by the Sovereign Military Order of Malta (SMOM) in collaboration with the German Leprosy Association and the Malta Government. The project was eventually approved by the World Health Organization. The project was led by Professor Enno Freerksen, Director of the Borstel Research Institute of Hamburg. Two Maltese physicians – Dr. George Depasquale and Dr Edgar Bonnici – were enrolled in the project, aided by Dr Anton Agius Ferrante. This project succeeded in eradicating Hansen disease as an endemic condition in the Maltese Islands.

Prevalence, Incidence & Hospital Statistics

Relevant Timeline

- 1893: publication of Ordinance No. VII entitled *An Ordinance for checking the spread of the disease commonly known as Leprosy*.
- 1900: opening in Malta of first residential leprosarium for males
- 1912. residential services in Malta extended for females.
- 1937: opening in Gozo of residential services for males and females.
- 1953: Act XI repealing of a large part of Lepers Ordinance abolishing compulsory internment except under special circumstances.
- 1972: initiation of the Leprosy Eradication project.

Incidence & Prevalence figures

Year	Population	year reported	Number notified			Leprosy incidence per 100,000 pop	Number known cases			Leprosy prevalence per 100,000 pop
			Male	Female	Total		Male	Female	Total	
1900										
1901	202134				4	1.98				
1902	205059				3	1.46				
1903	206689				8	3.87				
1904	209974				6	2.86				
1905	212888				7	3.29				
1906	215879				2	0.93				
1907	213395				4	1.87				
1908	215332				4	1.86				
1909	216617				5	2.31				
1910	216879				4	1.84				
1911	218542				9	4.12				
1912	220968				5	2.26				
1913	223741				20	8.94				
1914	224323				20	8.92				
1915	224655				21	9.35				
1916	224859				15	6.67				
1917	226224				13	5.75				
1918	215439				9	4.18				
1919	218510				2	0.92				
1920	220060				21	9.54				
1921	223088				16	7.17				
1922	225242	1925			14	6.22				
1923	227440				11	4.84				
1924	228575				12	5.25				
1925	230618				17	7.37				
1926	232832				16	6.87				
1927	234454				13	5.54				
1928	237782				15	6.31				
1929	247338				16	6.47				

Year	Population	year reported	Number notified			Leprosy incidence per 100,000 pop	Number known cases			Leprosy prevalence per 100,000 pop
			Male	Female	Total		Male	Female	Total	
1930	251846	1932			18	7.15				
1931	255197	1932			13	5.09				
1932	256140	1933			17	6.64				
1933	262165	1934			12	4.58				
1934	264663	1935			8	3.02				
1935	268668	1936			23	8.56				
1936	269912	1937			22	8.15				
1937	270755	1938			14	5.17				
1938	272359	1939			23	8.44				
1939	269090		7	5	12	4.46				
1940	272121		5	8	13	4.78				
1941	279187	1943	11	9	20	7.16				
1942	286596	1943	6	5	11	3.84				
1943	295247	1945	13	10	23	7.79				
1944	303998	1947	6	4	10	3.29				
1945	308929	1948	6	9	15	4.86				
1946	312722	1948	0	4	4	1.28				
1947	312447	1949	10	3	13	4.16				
1948	312600	1949	7	7	14	4.48	71	61	132	42.23
1949	314907	1950	10	5	15	4.76	81	56	137	43.50
1950	317248	1951	6	6	12	3.78	88	59	147	46.34
1951	319787	1953	4	1	5	1.56	93	59	152	47.53
1952	314066	1954	9	5	14	4.46	101	65	166	52.86
1953	319668	1954	6	5	11	3.44	92	61	153	47.86
1954	321940	1956	10	0	10	3.11	94	60	154	47.84
1955	324842	1956	6	8	14	4.31	90	60	150	46.18
1956	328854	1958	12	7	19	5.78	89	59	148	45.00
1957	329011	1959	13	8	21	6.38	94	57	151	45.90
1958	328854	1961	7	8	15	4.56	104	64	168	51.09
1959	329001	1961	9	6	15	4.56				0.00
1960	328116	1962	6	3	9	2.74			132	40.23
1961	323591	1968	10	4	14	4.33	112	70	182	56.24
1962	319164	1969	1	2	3	0.94	113	74	187	58.59
1963	317482	1969			13	4.09	118	79	197	62.05
1964	318573	1969			11	3.45	121	80	201	63.09
1965	302218	1970			16	5.29	128	80	208	68.82
1966	302486	1970			10	3.31	128	82	210	69.42
1967	302820	1970			12	3.96	128	84	212	70.01
1968	303161				8	2.64	134	81	215	70.92
1969	303114				8	2.64	134	85	219	72.25
1970	302219				7	2.32	139	83	222	73.46
1971	301892				6	1.99	139	86	225	74.53
1972	306551				4	1.30	138	86	224	73.07
1973	311150				8	2.57				
1974	315466				5	1.58				
1975	318320				7	2.20				
1976	322535				5	1.55				
1977	325721				1	0.31				
1978	328375				2	0.61				
1979	331859				2	0.60				
1980	335169				2	0.60				
1981	338276				1	0.30				
1982	340907				4	1.17				

Year	Population	year reported	Number notified			Leprosy incidence per 100,000 pop	Number known cases			Leprosy prevalence per 100,000 pop
			Male	Female	Total		Male	Female	Total	
1983	343334				1	0.29				
1984	345636				0	0.00				
1985	345705				4	1.16				
1986	348372				3	0.86				
1987	350914				5	1.42				
1988	354532				2	0.56				
1989	358188				3	0.84				
1990	361908				0	0.00				
1991	365781				0	0.00				
1992	369455				1	0.27				
1993	373161				1	0.27				
1994	376433				0	0.00				
1995	378404				0	0.00				
1996	381405				0	0.00				
1997	384176				1	0.26				
1998	386397				0	0.00			85	22.00
1999	388759				0	0.00			84	21.61
2000	391415				1	0.26			72	18.39
2001	394641				0	0.00			69	17.48
2002	397296				0	0.00			70	17.62
2003	399867				0	0.00			68	17.01
2004	402668				0	0.00			66	16.39
2005	404999				0	0.00			61	15.06
2006	405616				0	0.00			57	14.05
2007	407832				0	0.00			57	13.98
2008	410926				0	0.00			50	12.17
2009	414027				0	0.00			47	11.35
2010	414989				0	0.00	29	14	43	10.36
2011	417546				0	0.00	28	14	42	10.06
2012	422509				0	0.00	24	12	36	8.52
2013	429424				0	0.00	23	10	33	7.68
2014	439691				0	0.00	23	11	34	7.73
2015	450415				0	0.00	21	11	32	7.10
2016	460297				0	0.00	19	10	29	6.30
2017	467999				0	0.00	19	9	28	5.98
2018	484630				0	0.00	18	6	24	4.95
2019	502653				1	0.21			23	4.58
2020	515000				0	0.00			21	4.08

Hospital Prevalence

Year	Population	Malta Institution			Gozo institution			Hospital Prevalence per 100,000 pop
		Male	Female	Total	Male	Female	Total	
1900		69		69				34.50 *[approximate]*
1901	202134	63		63				31.17
1902	205059	62		62				30.24
1903	206689	60		60				29.03
1904	209974	62		62				29.53
1905	212888	65		65				30.53
1906	215879	63		63				29.18
1907	213395	66		66				30.93
1908	215332	65		65				30.19
1909	216617	60		60				27.70
1910	216879	58		58				26.74
1911	218542	57		57				26.08
1912	220968	54	36	90				40.73
1913	223741	63	44	107				47.82
1914	224323	62	45	107				47.70
1915	224655	63	42	105				46.74
1916	224859	66	40	106				47.14
1917	226224	67	38	105				46.41
1918	215439	69	35	104				48.27
1919	218510	61	32	93				42.56
1920	220060	51	30	81				36.81
1921	223088	46	31	77				34.52
1922	225242	45	26	71				31.52
1923	227440	45	28	73				32.10
1924	228575	40	27	67				29.31
1925	230618	32	23	55				23.85
1926	232832	37	25	62				26.63
1927	234454	37	32	69				29.43
1928	237782	41	29	70				29.44
1929	247338	41	31	72				29.11
1930	251846	46	25	71				28.19
1931	255197	43	24	67				26.25
1932	256140	42	25	67				26.16
1933	262165	39	21	60				22.89
1934	264663	36	57	93				35.14
1935	268668	53	23	76				28.29
1936	269912	55	24	79	*Sacred Heart Hospital opened*			29.27
1937	270755	43	25	68	13	2	15	30.66
1938	272359	51	29	80	13	2	15	34.88
1939	269090	49	26	75	14	4	18	34.56
1940	272121	43	22	65	16	4	20	31.24
1941	279187	43	27	70	16	7	23	33.31
1942	286596			68			21	31.05
1943	295247			69			18	29.47
1944	303998			71			17	28.95
1945	308929			74	11	6	17	29.46
1946	312722			73	9	6	15	28.14
1947	312447			70	8	7	15	27.20
1948	312600	43	23	66	7	8	15	25.91
1949	314907	52	29	81	4	6	10	28.90
1950	317248	58	31	89	6	7	13	32.15
1951	319787	63	32	95	6	7	13	33.77
1952	314066	66	37	103	6	7	13	36.93

Year	Population	Malta Institution			Gozo institution			Hospital Prevalence per 100,000 pop
		Male	Female	Total	Male	Female	Total	
1953	319668	54	21	75	3	5	8	25.96
1954	321940	53	19	72	3	3	6	24.23
1955	324842	50	20	70	3	0	3	22.47
1956	328854	28	12	40			0	12.16
1957	329011	29	14	43	*Sacred Heart Hospital closed*			13.07
1958	328854	29	14	43				13.08
1959	329001	29	14	43				13.07
1960	328116	26	13	39				11.89
1961	323591	26	15	41				12.67
1962	319164	27	17	44				13.79
1963	317482	23	19	42				13.23
1964	318573	24	18	42				13.18
1965	302218	24	18	42				13.90
1966	302486	23	17	40				13.22
1967	302820	22	16	38				12.55
1968	303161	23	17	40				13.19
1969	303114	24	17	41				13.53
1970	302219	24	17	41				13.57
1971	301892	24	17	41				13.58
1972	306551	24	17	41				13.37
1973	311150							
1974	315466			22				6.97
1975	318320	*St. Bartholomew Hospital closed*						
1976	322535	*Hal Ferha estate opened*						
1977	325721							
1978	328375							
1979	331859							
1980	335169							
1981	338276							
1982	340907							
1983	343334							
1984	345636							
1985	345705							
1986	348372							
1987	350914			6				1.71
1988	354532							
1989	358188							
1990	361908							
1991	365781							
1992	369455							
1993	373161							
1994	376433	3	2	5				1.33
1995	378404	3	2	5				1.32
1996	381405			4				1.05
1997	384176			4				1.04
1998	386397			4				1.04
1999	388759			2				0.51
2000	391415			1				0.26
2001	394641			1				0.25
2002	397296			0				0.00
2003	399867			0				0.00
2004	402668			0				0.00
2005	404999	*Hal Ferha estate closed*						

St. Bartholomew's Hospital – patient movement

Year	Admitted	Transferred from other hospitals	Transferred to other hospital	Discharged at request	Cured	Relieved	Died	Remaining end year
1900	81	0	0	0	0	0	12	69
1901	4	0	0	0	0	0	10	63
1902	3	0	0	0	0	0	4	62
1903	2	0	0	0	0	0	4	60
1904	6	0	0	0	0	0	4	62
1905	6	0	0	0	0	0	3	65
1906	1	0	0	0	0	0	3	63
1907	4	0	0	0	0	0	1	66
1908	4	0	0	0	2	0	3	65
1909	4	0	0	1	0	0	8	60
1910	3	0	0	0	0	0	5	58
1911	10	0	0	0	0	0	11	57
1912	41	0	0	0	0	0	8	90
1913	29	0	0	0	0	0	12	107
1914	18	0	0	0	3	0	15	107
1915	11	0	0	0	0	0	13	105
1916	14	0	0	0	2	0	11	106
1917	18	0	0	0	1	0	18	105
1918	10	0	0	1	0	0	10	104
1919	9	0	0	0	9	0	11	93
1920	9	0	0	0	10	0	11	81
1921	4	0	0	0	1	0	7	77
1922	5	0	0	1	4	0	6	71
1923	13	0	0	1	0	0	10	73
1924	8	0	0	0	2	0	12	67
1925	4	0	0	0	10	0	6	55
1926	15	0	0	0	0	0	8	62
1927	12	0	0	0	1	0	4	69
1928	13	0	0	1	1	0	10	70
1929	11	0	0	1	0	0	8	72
1930	17	0	0	3	1	0	10	71
1931	7	0	0	0	0	0	11	67
1932	12	0	0	0	2	0	10	67
1933	9	0	0	0	2	0	14	60
1934	6	0	0	0	2	0	7	93
1935	21	0	0	0	0	0	2	76
1936	20	0	0	0	3	0	14	77
1937	16	0	15	0	4	0	6	68
1938	23	0	0	0	2	0	9	80
1939	6	0	0	0	8	0	6	75
1940	7	0	3	0	6	0	8	65
1941	18	0	2	0	1	0	10	70
1942	10	0	0	0	4	0	11	68
1943	17	0	0	0	3	0	13	69
1944	12	0	0	0	1	0	9	71
1945	10	0	0	0	3	0	4	74
1946	7	0	0	0	3	0	5	73
1947	10	0	0	0	2	0	11	70
1948	9	0	0	0	2	0	11	66
1949	20	0	0	0	1	0	4	81
1950	11	0	0	1	1	0	1	89
1951	6	1	0	0	0	0	1	95
1952	14	0	0	1	2	0	3	103
1953	6	2	1	31	0	0	4	75
1954	7	0	0	6	0	0	4	72
1955	4	1	0	3	0	0	4	70
1956	11	0	0	36	0	0	5	40
1957	12	1	0	7	0	0	3	43
1958	2	0	0	2	0	0	0	43
1959	4	0	0	2	0	0	2	43
1960	2	0	0	0	0	1	5	39
1961	5	0	0	0	0	0	3	41

Cont.

Year	Admitted	Transferred from other hospitals	Transferred to other hospital	Discharged at request	Cured	Relieved	Died	Remaining end year
1962	6	0	0	0	0	0	3	44
1963	3	0	0	3	0	0	2	42
1964	3	0	0	3	0	0	2	42
1965	3	0	0	2	0	0	2	42
1966	0	0	0	1	0	0	2	42
1967	0	0	0	0	0	0	2	42
1968	3	0	0	0	0	0	1	42
1969	2	0	0	0	0	0	1	42
1970	2	0	0	0	0	0	2	42
1971	1	0	0	0	0	0	1	42
1972	0	0	0	0	0	0	2	39

Sacred Heart Hospital – patient movement

Year	Admitted	Transferred from other hospitals	Transferred to other hospital	Discharged at request	Cured	Relieved	Died	Remaining end year
1938	1	0	0	0	0	0	1	15
1939	4	0	0	0	0	0	1	18
1940	0	3	0	0	0	0	1	20
1941	3	2	0	0	0	0	2	23
1942	1	0	0	0	0	0	1	23
1943	4	0	0	0	2	0	4	21
1944	0	0	0	0	0	0	3	18
1945	0	0	0	0	0	0	1	17
1946	0	0	0	0	0	0	2	15
1947	1	0	0	0	0	0	1	15
1948	1	0	0	0	0	0	1	15
1949	0	0	0	0	0	2	3	10
1950	4	0	0	0	0	0	1	13
1951	1	0	1	0	0	0	0	13
1952	1	1	1	0	0	0	1	13
1953	0	0	2	1	0	0	3	8
1954	0	0	1	1	0	0	0	6
1955	0	0	1	2	0	0	0	3
1956	1	0	1	2	0	0	1	0

Annotated Bibliography

A: Archives – Manuscript sources

1. *Registrum Fundationum Beneficiorum Insulae Gaudisii*. Ms. Malta Archiepiscopal Archives, f.59-59v (24.iii.1492). Transcribed in: Busuttil J. Fiorini S, editors. Documentary Sources of Maltese history. Part V Documents in the Curia of the Archbishop of Malta. No. 1 The Registrum Fundationum Beneficiorum Insulae Gaudisii 1435-1545. University Press, Malta, 2006, doc.57, 80-81.

    - Describes the first documented case of leprosy termed *erga corpore morbo lepre* is said to have affected a Gozitan woman Garita Xejbais who bequeathed land in the district of Ghajn Xejba to the Church in 1492.

    Die vigesimo quarto martii X indictionis millesimo quartigentesimo nongesimo primo // ... //
    Testamur quod Garita puella quondam Nardi Xeiba, **erga corpore morbo lepre***, sana tamen mente et rationis compos existens, presentibus testibus infrascriptis per me notarium Jacobum Sabbara procuravit facere presentem codicillum, et sic legavit Ecclesie Gloriose Virginis Marie contrate Hajn Xeibe medietatem pro indiviso unius pecie terre aratorie que dicitur Nighered, site et posite in eadem contrata, cuius reliqua medietas est Nicolai de Nastasio, confinate cum terris Masi Zabbar et Pauli de Girardo ac Antonii de Bernardo et hoc ut de eius fructibus serviatur marammati et luminariis dicte ecclesie, videlicet, in incedendo lamadem vel lumeram quolibet sero Sabbati Paschatis et Natalis Domini Nostri Jesu Κριστι et festivitabus eiusdem ecclesie ac etian [f.59ᵛ] in conficiendo pane duorum thumenorum frumenti distribuendo, more Gaudisii, personis qui in festivitate dicte ecclesie interfuerint et celebrari facirndo unam Missam in eadem festivitate ac etiam constituit, ordinavit et fecit in eius fidei commissarium huius rei sive procuratorem, gubernatorem et administratorem dictorum fructuum Angelum de Marino, substituendo, post eiusdem Angeli decessum, Johannem filium eiusdem Angeli et Laurentium utique filium eiusdem Angeli. Quem codicillum mandavit servari per eius heredes et valeat per m[odum quo] melius valere potest, tam iure codicillorum quam cuiusvis alterius ultime volluntatis // ... //*
    <Tenor autem testamentorum, codicillorum et aliorum actorum ad pias causas legatorum ex actis, registris, prothocollis et thecis quondam egregii Guillelimi Sanso notarii publici extractorum sequitur et est talis, videlicet: In nomine Domini Amen. Anno Dominice Incarnationis millesimo quadragentesimo nongesimo quinto mense Februarii decimo eiusdem mensis XIII inditionis, regnante Serenissimo // ... //

2. National Malta Library [NML]: *Domini Sanatatis Manuscript 153*, fol. 421; *Manuscript 740*, fol. 36t – as reported by P. Cassar, 1965, 210.

    - Documents the public health laws of the OSJ promulgated in Rhodes aiming to limit the spread of the disease. The "sick of Saint Lazarus" were beneficiaries of special charities from the Order and cared for in their homes. These regulations debarred infected individuals from having any social intercourse with healthy ones who in turn were prohibited under penalty of a hefty fine from receiving any goods from lepers. Furthermore, lepers were precluded from practicing certain occupations unless licensed by the sanitary authorities who ensured that material goods belonging to lepers was not physically passed on to healthy people.

3. Archives of the Dominican Priory, Rabat (Malta): *De statu trium conventum.* Parte I, f.129t, 188 – as reported by P. Cassar, *The Medical History of Malta.* Wellcome Historical Medical Library, London, 1965, 210

   - Describes a case of leprosy in Malta involving a Dominican friar who died in the Rabat convent in Malta in 1629. Entry records how on the 1 July 1629 the Priory of St. Dominic of rabat bought a 'white slave for sixty ounces, called Bacher, from Castelnuovo' to attend to the needs of the friar who dies a leper on the 30 April 1630.

4. NML: *Commissione perche provedesse ai poveri affetti dal terribile morbo della lebra. Liber Concilium Archives of the Order of Malta [AOM] 121,* f.53 – as reported by P. Cassar, 1965, 210-211.

   - On 29 October 1659, the Council of the Order voices concern about the fate of the sick poor suffering from leprosy.

5. NML: *AOM 262,* f.97, 141 – as reported by P. Cassar, 1965, 210-211.

   - Documents the 21 March 1679 recommendations of the *Commissione* appointed to inquire into the management of the hospital services proposing that foreign lepers who had no relatives in Malta to look after them were to be housed in that part of the *Sacra Infermeria* known as the *Falanga* which was reserved for patients suffering from 'contagious' diseases. Before alleged lepers were admitted into the infirmary, they were examined by the whole medical and surgical staff of the hospital in the presence of the Venerab;e Hospitaller, the infirmarian and the 'prud-hommes' to ascertain that the disease was really leprosy. In case of lepers living in Malta, no in-patient treatment was considered necessary by the Commissionn; on the contrary it was suggested that they should be granted financial aid and retained in their homes. The Council approved the recommendations.

6. *Status Animarum II : 1687* – as reported by S. Fiorini. Proceedings of History Week 1984, University Press, Malta, 1986, 41-100.

   - Reports one case of leprosy in the population

Condition	Locality	Sex	Age	Description/Remarks
Leprosy	Qormi, Malta	F	30	*Maritus (28) non cohabitat*

7. G. Demarco: *Tractatus affectuum cutaneorum NML Manuscript 36,* 1764, n.p.

   - This theses about cutaneous disorders includes a chapter on leprosy.

8. NML: *Manuscript 1146bis*, f.74, 1770-72
   - A contemporary diary reports the occurrence of leprosy in a nun in the Monastery of St. Catherine in Valletta, Malta who on 21 October 1770 'developed ulcers and fever and also became leprous' to die three weeks later; and the arrival to Malta on 15 May 1772 of the son of a Turkish high official on his way to Montpellier accompanied by his personal Greek physician to seek a cure there.

9. Medical & Health Archives: *Letters to Government from 20 April 1888 to 8 April 1895*. f.300, 515, 550, 611, 639 – as reported in P. Cassar, 1965, 213-215
   - Reports that in a population survey was conducted in 1890 to assess the size of the problem, only 69 known cases of leprosy were identified suggesting a prevalence rate of 42 per 100,000 population; eight of which lived in Gozo – four from Nadur. Only eleven cases were in an advanced stage of the disease and had admitted themselves to the Asylum for the Aged and Incurables, commonly known as the Poor House. The rest were scattered in different parts of the Islands – the greater number of cases in Malta came from rural areas, mainly Qormi and Mosta, only one came from Valletta; eight came from Gozo, four of whom from Nadur. Of those victims living at home, nine were willing to be admitted into the asylum but this could not accommodate them. Some of those living in the community had occupations considered risky for the rest of the community – baker, pasta maker, cook, milkman and shopkeeper. Proposal was made to legislate on lines as other legislation existing in other British colonies to control the spread of the infection [f.300].
   - Subsequent correspondence proposed the conversion into a leprosarium of Selmun Tower or the large house on Comino – both premises were however considered too small [f.639].
   - Also reports the various episodes of disturbances caused by the lepers on 24 May 1900 and September 1900 when the police had to intervene to restore order [f.515, 550, 611].

10. Medical & Health Archives: *Letters to Government from 10 April 1895 to 31 March 1903*. f.534; *Letters to Government from 1 April 1903 to 10 April 1909*. f.4, 36, 48, 611 – as reported in P. Cassar, 1965, 215-216
    - Proposal to make escape from the leprosarium a criminal offence with escapee being liable to imprisonment for a period ranging from 1-6 months [1895-1903, f.534.; 1903-1909, f.48]
    - Reports the introduction of the measure of employing young able-bodied patients for household duties with a small monthly remuneration [1903-1909, f.4, 611].
    - Asylum attendant granted police powers; six armed constables under a sergeant were employed for night duties [1903-1909, f.36].

11. Medical & Health Archives: *Visitors' Book – Leper Hospital, Malta.* – as reported by the *Reports on Workings of Government Department …. during 1930-31*, 1932, R9.
    - Entry dated 21 October 1930: H.H. Lieutenant-Governor – "I visited the wards of the Poor House, as well as the Leper Hospital, and am much impressed both by the size of the former Institution and by the excellent condition in which both appear to be kept".

- Entry dated 23 January 1931: H.E. the Governor – "The operation of the new law has not yet resulted in a reduction in the number of lepers under treatment in the Leper Hospital. I was informed that there are three out-patients attending the hospital for treatment and that the policy of inspecting contacts with new cases is resented by the contacts themselves. I hope that every effort will be made to explain to these people that this inspection is made in their own interests as well as those of the Community and I also hope that the unpopularity of the measure will not lead to any relaxation".

B: Published Case reports

1. G. Gulia: Sopra un caso di Lebbra dei Greci. *Il Barth : gazzetta di medicina e scienze naturali*, 29 January 1874, 3(19):372-377

    - Reports three cases – two under the case of Prof. Schinas diagnosed circa 1835, and one discussed in detail seen by author circa 1874.
    - Reports that Dr. Gerlach believed that the Medieval *hospitalis Sanctj Franciscj*, situated outside the Medieval walls of Mdina, had been initially established as a leprosarium.

Sopra un caso di lebbra dei Greci.

Una delle più formidabili malattie, a cui è soggetta l'umana famiglia, è la lebbra, non senza ragione dagli Indiani chiamata il *male* per antonomasia. " Essa " dice Areteo, che con molta maestria la descrive " venne anche appellata *morbo erculeo*, come il più poderoso e il maggiore di tutti i morbi."

Circa dodici anni addietro il nostro Governo sceglieva una commissione di medici per rispondere ad alcuni quesiti che gli si dirigevano dal Collegio medico di Londra, allora occupato della distribuzione geografica di codesta infermità: e la conchiusione ne fu che nissun caso di lebbra essendosi mai offerto alla osservazione di quei medici, nè dei loro contemporanei, tale morbo doveasi considerare estraneo a quest'isola. Membro di quel comitato anch'io vi annuiva, quantunque oggi io pensi diversamente; imperocchè inseguito fui informato che nel 1835 ricoveravasi nella clinica del prof. Schinas, un lebbroso giunto agli estremi periodi del morbo; e mi si parlò di un individuo di 55 anni, morto or non pochi anni di *psoriasi con artrite*, nel quale si erano manifestate varie deformazioni scheletriche, il che mi fa molto dubitare della esattezza della diagnosi. A me stesso inoltre si è ultimamente presentato un infermo di lebbra, che da altri fu considerato e trattato per podagroso, il che non deve recar gran sorpresa, poichè trattandosi di un morbo proteiforme, come è la lebbra massime al suo esordire, non è difficile che inciampino in errori di diagnosi medici non attaccati allo studio nè all'osservazione o che non l'anno studiato in clinica o nei paesi ove regna endemico. Infatti lo Schilling, che ci ha lasciato una dissertazione classica intorno a cotesta affezione, così scrive: " *perdifficile est ejus principium cognoscere, et prima pullulantis mali signa observare:"* e Heberden assevera che questa infermità spesso rimane per anni limitata ad una o due macchie gialle, persistenti ed indelebili alla parte interna ed inferiore delle gambe. Laonde io credo che di quando in quando se ne avveri qui qualche caso che venga riferito ad affesioni artritiche, erpetiche, sifilitiche e simili: lo stesso Collegio medico di Londra, non ostante la relazione suddetta, menziona quest'isola fra i luoghi, dove tuttavia la lebbra si manifesta.

Nata nell'Affrica cocente, la lebbra fece il gran giro del globo: invase l'Italia e tutta Europa quando Roma avea sottoposto tutto l'Oriente. Comune altrevolte da noi, massime all'epoca della dominazione araba, essa è qui conosciuta col suo nome arabo di *Gidiem*. Il dott. Gerlach, che visitava questa isola ora sono pochi anni, crede che l'Ospedale Santo Spirito, uno dei più antichi di Europa, sia stato istituito pei lebbrosi. Fortunatamente cotesta terribile egritudine è divenuta tanto rara in Europa che la comparsa di un caso vi si nota come una curiosità patologica: occasionalmente se ne sviluppa qualche caso in Creta, Cefalonia, Grecia, Russia, Svezia, Norvegia, Irlanda, nelle coste settentrionali d'Italia, e nelle regioni sud-orientali della Francia, in Spagna e nel Portogallo: ma sfortunatamente sono tuttavia vastissime regioni afflitte dalla lebbra, che nell'Asia Minore, e nelle Indie Orientali conta a migliaia le sue vittime.

Il caso da me non ha guari osservato è molto interessante, e però offrendone ai lettori di questa effemeride una descrizione, credo far loro cosa grata. La lebbra od elefantiasi dei Greci, essendo, come ho detto, proteiforme, è conosciuta dagli autori sotto varie denominazioni, se ne distinguono due principali varietà, la tubercolosa e la bianca o non tubercolosa. A quest'ultima, detta *leuce* o *lebbra alfoide*, si riferisce il seguente caso.

N.N. di temperamento bilioso-nervoso, fino all'età di 28 anni, compiti l'anno 1850, aveva sempre goduto un'intera e perfetta salute. Passò una gioventù briosa fra il canto e il suono; ma parco nel bere e di onesti costumi non si era mai dato al vizio, e non ebbe perciò mali sifilitici, tampoco una semplice blenorragia. Esperto suonatore di chitarra, egli ne accompagnava il suono con dolce canto, traendosi dietro, specialmente le sere d'estate, numerosa caterva di giovani. L'anno 1850, alla seconda epidemia colerica, morì sua madre; e, parte pel dolore e parte pel timore panico, patì vari sconcerti nervosi ai quali egli faceva risalire la sua malattia. Che il suo carattere cominciasse d'allora a mutarsi, l'indicava la chitarra che o taceva, oppur mossa da umori malinconici accompagnava qualche strofetta religiosa che più non allettava le turbe giovanili. Poco a poco andò egli riducendosi ad una vita ritirata, e finì per darsi in preda alla più profonda malinconia. Le uniche gioje che provasse da quinci innanzi gli erano ispirate dal sentimento religioso, che in lui andò sempre più sviluppandosi. Nell'inverno del 1850 soffrì un freddo insolito, e s'avvide di un'eruzione al braccio destro, di macchie rosee che cuoprivansi di squammette di color argentino perlato: gli arti toracici, gli addominali, il tronco e la faccia, mano mano divennero la sede di tale eruzione. Coteste macchie andavano aumentando in numero, ed alcune crescevano in area, per la qual cosa molte insieme si confondevano, occupandogli così un vasto territorio della pelle. La eruzione produceva un prurito che talora era così considerabile da obbligare il malato a grattarsi con impeto e produrre abrasioni; questo prurito spesso gli impediva il sonno. Alcuni scrittori medioevali, che ci danno la più ampia descrizione della lebbra, si occuparono molto di cotesto prurito; *ac si acubus pugantur, aut urtica percussi essent aut vermibus roderentur*. La pelle attaccata eprimevasi alquanto, ma non in tutte le macchie; più in quelle degli arti superiori che degli inferiori. Tale fenomeno non isfuggì all'autore del Levitico, il quale dice che "i tegumenti in questi egri non conservano il medesimo livello." Altronde è noto come i Libri Santi traccino con dipintura raffaellesca questa maravigliosa degenerazione del sistema umano, come la chiama l'Alibert, la quale era l'infermità colla quale il Signore avea visitato vari personaggi bibblici, tali sono Faraone, Naaman e Miriam.

Intanto, quantunque le scaglie si rimuovessero facilmente coll'olio di oliva e colla glicerina, pure esse si rinnovavano presto. Verso gli ultimi anni di sua vita tutto l'ambito della cute era preso dalla eruzione, la quale a misura che acquistava territorio andava suscitando una dispnea sempre più forte. L'estate del 1856 cominciò a molestarlo un dolore nelle articolazioni delle dita, e un anno dopo si vide comparire tumefazioni in varie regioni della pelle: poscia brutte contrazioni ed ingorghi, dimostranti l'alterazione del tessuto cellulare, gli si manifestarono nei piedi e nelle mani: le gambe si ingrossarono come fossero edematose: nei ginocchi si stabilì un gonfiore che non permetteva più la flessione delle gambe: le dita della mano si assottigliarono per atrofia dei loro muscoli e si mantenevano riflesse per evidente accorciamento dei tendini flessori: le unghia si contorsero in varie guise, alcune si annerirono e divennero adunche ed acute di modo che la mano sembrava la gamba di un uccello di rapina: essa avea perduto quella squisita sensibilità che le ha procurato il nome di secondo cervello. *Articuli eorum sunt nodosi et distorti, ungues lividi ed incurvi.* A cagione dei quali disordini da quattro anni egli camminava barcollando, e provava grandissima difficoltà per salire le scale; pure, come tutti i lebbrosi, si ingegnava di uscire di casa quasi giornalmente e recavasi in chiesa, dove stava parecchie ore. Intanto al principio del 1871 alcune ulcerette gli si aprirono sullo stinco sinistro, le quali in una sola si fusero che rendeva una sanie abbondante e purulenta. Accusava spesso una irritazione alla laringe e di quando in quando la voce era rauca ed aveva un suono nasale: *vox clangosa et rauca, et interdum ægri per nares quasi videntur loqui.* È noto da quanto ci narra San Luca come i dieci lebbrosi portati innanzi a N. S. fossero tosto riconosciuti dal suono della loro voce. Ma questi disturbi vocali nel mio ammalato non erano dipendenti da vizi organici, come spesso avviene nei lebbrosi, sibbene da causa nervosa, imperocchè non erano continui, di guisa che la voce spesso riprendeva tutta la sonorità normale.

Anchilosi e contorsioni simili alle suddescritte non risparmiarono alcuna parte del corpo. In sui da otto anni i movimenti del collo s'andavano rendendo più difficili, finchè verso il 1870 divennero del tutto impossibili, di guisa che l'infermo si rivolgeva tutto un pezzo. La respirazione era addominale, poichè anche le articolazioni costo-spinali eransi tumefatte in modo da impedire i movimenti respiratori del torace. La faccia era di color terreo e spesso livida. Lo avresti detto una perfetta mummia a cui solo gli occhi dessero segno di vita: e ti avrebbe rammentato il caso di Miriam che era come morto. Ebbe adunque ben ragione il Depons quando disse che questo male attenta meno alla esistenza dell'uomo, che alle sue forme, che esso faccia consistere il suo trionfo più nel degenerarlo che nel distruggerlo, quantunque esso poi dopo anni finisca per troncargli la misera esistenza. Uno dei sintomi più costanti nell'infermo era la coprostasi, che talora dosi ripetute di purganti non valevano a vincere. Anche Areteo fa menzione di cotesto fenomeno. Le cilia gli si erano allungate come succede spesso nei bambini scrofolosi; i peli non cadevano da tutte le macchie; ma l'alopecia verso gli ultimi mesi già cominciava a manifestarsi nella testa che era la meno colpita dalla degenerazione lebbrosa. Nell'estate del 1872 cominciò a manifestarsi un gonfiore edematoso negli organi genitali che molto si erano sfigurati; e le gambe, già ipertrofizzate, anch'esse divennero edematose. Nel settembre del 1872, un versamento idropico gli si verificava nel ventre, e nel dicembre dell'anno seguente ebbe compiuto anasarca. Il respiro affannoso ed altri sintomi accennavano ad un edema polmonale. Cotesti versamenti idropici non sembravano provenire da disturbi nefritici o epatici, nè da vizi valvolari, imperocchè mancava ogni sintoma di affezione renale epatica e cardiaca; essi erano dipendenti da un'anemia, di cui erano manifesti tutti i caratteri. La digitale aveva trionfato per qualche tempo delle infiltrazioni, ma perchè l'aglobulia era invincibile, gli edemi ritornarono presto. Un sintomo curioso e, secondo lo Schilling ed alcuni moderni scrittori, costante della lebbra, era la disturbata innervazione della cute e delle macchie, in alcune delle quali vi fu anestesia, in altre solo analgesia, in altre infine un'isterica iperestesia. È curioso a sapere come le macchie più piccole fossero circondate da un'aureola iperestesica. L'analgesia non era mai tale da impedire che l'egro sentisse l'introduzione d'un ago nella pelle. Un altro fenomeno degno di osservazione era un freddo continuo e talora così intenso da obbligare l'infermo anche nell'estate a cuoprirsi di lana: nei giorni della canicola le sue mani erano diaccie, e mentre ognuno si lamentava della grande arsura, egli solo si lagnava del freddo! segno evidente che il processo di ossidazione, sorgente del calore animale, si era molto diminuito nel suo organismo: " imperocchè dice Areteo " a tali infermi rado tocca di sortir un'ottima ed omogenea assimilazione."

Lungo il suo decorso, la malattia, quanto ai dolori ed all'eruzione, offriva esacerbazioni e remissioni: queste ultime avvenivano nell'estate, come si verifica in tutte le psoriasi e negli eczemi. L'uso degli arsenicali moderava alquanto l'eruzione, scolorendo le macchie; ma non sembrava esercitare alcuna azione sulle degenerazioni suddescritte.

Quanto alla psiche, io non credo che questo infermo l'abbia avuta integra: l'estrema tristezza, e l'ascetismo troppo spunto sarebbero stati bastevoli perchè io lo considerassi sotto l'impulso di idee deliranti, se una transitoria ma perfetta amenomania non fosse venuta a dimostrarmi colla maggiore evidenza che anche il suo cervello aveva comunque partecipato della degenerazione lebbrosa. Egli ebbe inoltre allucinazione della vista e dell'udito, avendo veduto il demonio in una figura minaccevole, che, comparsogli in una notte gli parlò poscia per vari giorni di seguito. La *libido inexplebilis* di alcuni lebbrosi non è che una leggiera monomania erotica, della quale l'infermo, di cui narro il caso, non presentò alcuna sintomia, soggiogato come fu dal sentimento ascetico. I vecchi lebbrosi che il Sonnini narra aver veduto darsi senza alcun pudore ai trasporti più disonesti in mezzo alle strade, avevano pur essi l'intelligenza perturbata: infatti alcuni si abbandonano col maggior impeto ad un congresso sessuale poche ore prima della morte. L'ascetismo avea ridotto il nostro infermo all'anafrodisia, e l'Alibert anch'egli riferisce la storia di un lebbroso che avea perduto la facoltà virile. Ciò non ostante in alcuni casi ciò che fa uscire il lebbroso dai limiti della decenza, si è un'ipertrofia degli organi genitali. Così lo Schilling narra di aver osservato un lebbroso la cui verga avea acquistato la lunghezza di oltre a sette piedi: nei quali casi si ha satiriasi anzichè monomania erotica. L'infermo, di cui espongo il caso, non presentò negli organi genitali nulla fuori delle macchie esulcerate, e dell'enfiagione edematosa alla quale ho più sopra accennato.

Intanto il marasmo era giunto al suo colmo: l'infermo non poteva più digerire il poco che mangiava. Nei primi di dicembre del 1873 la ulcera della gamba si disseccava, e quindi gli sopravvenne una diarrea incoercibile, la quale fece poco a poco sparire l'anasarca. La prostrazione era somma; il polso debole e depresso; la voce sepolcrale; quando in mezzo ad una grave ambascia la morte gli venne a porre fine alle lunghe e terribili sofferenze.

La causa che produsse in questo individuo la lebbra, è certamente un mistero. Egli non visse nell'immondezza, nè nella indigenza, nè in cattiva casa. Quanto alla eredità nulla posso asserire: egli mi parlò di un suo antenato che avrebbe avuto un'affezione simile, ma questa informazione mi fu data in modo diverso da altri membri della sua famiglia. Come la massima parte delle dermatosi squammose, questa infermità non sembra propagarsi per contagio; tale è almeno l'opinione di Van Someren, una delle più grandi autorità viventi intorno alla malattia in parola.

Quanto alla farmacia ci fu poco da fare. Il dottor Cannon, reduce da Gerusalemme dove erasi recato a studiare i lebbrosi, ebbe sotto sua cura per qualche tempo il suddetto infermo, a cui somministrò gli arsenicali coi risultati già menzionati. Van Someren che dirige nel Madras uno spedale di lebbrosi, loda l'alimentazione ricca, che anche i medici medioevali commendavano; e l'uso dell'olio dell'*Anacardium occidentale*, già adoperato nell'India contro varie dermatosi ribelli.

2. I. Sammut: Le Lebbre dei Greci. *Il Barth : gazzetta di medicina e scienze naturali*, 4 April 1874, 3(20):399-400

- Reports a number of cases from Malta – managed by Dr. V. Pirotta and Dr. Lanzon. A number of cases were also recorded in one particular family group.

La lebbra dei Greci.

Pubblichiamo con piacere la seguente notizia inviataci dal Sig. dott. I. Sammut, intorno alla lebbra dei Greci.

Siamo pure informati dal Sig. dott. V. Pirotti, che nella Vittoriosa trovasi da tempo una donna affetta dalla elefanziasi dei Greci: anche il sig. dott. Lanzon c'informa di un lebbroso, morto l'anno passato a Casal Luca, in cui questa terribile dermatosi si manifestò assai più grave che nell'infermo di cui nella precedente dispensa abbiamo dato la storia. Ciò dimostra quanto errasse quella giunta di medici che asseverava tale malattia essere estranea alla popolazione di quest'isola.

Nel No. 19 del *Barth*, ragionando della elefanziasi dei Greci, V. S. sostiene, contro l'opinione emessa da un comitato di medici pochi anni addietro, tale malattia non doversi considerare estranea a quest'isola. I fatti seguenti dimostrano che ella ha ragione, e che sufficienti indagini non si erano fatte, quando s'asseriva il contrario. Infatti dal 1839 al 1858 tutti i maschi di una famiglia nominata *Piscopo*, morirono di lebbra dopo averne sofferto per lunga serie di anni. È veramente curioso come le femmine ne sieno rimaste incolumi. Il primo ad essere colpito fu *Vincenzo*, che di anni 27 cessava di vivere il 6 marzo 1839, sotto cura dei medici A. Muscat e A. Gauci. Indi infermò *Giovanni*, che ne morì il 14 aprile 1847, in età di anni 32. Un fratello di costoro moriva anch'egli di elefanziasi il 12 giugno 1858; poco prima soccombeva il loro padre nella grave età di anni 72, cioè addì 24 nov. 1857, dopo penose e lunghe sofferenze. Oltre a questi ultimi tre ammalati, che essendo rimasti lungo tempo sotto mia cura, mi porsero ottima occasione perchè io osservassi la terribile infermità in parola, ne vidi altri casi in due sorelle reduci dall'Isola San Domingo, nelle quali, pochi anni dopo il loro arrivo in Malta, cominciò a manifestarsi la lebbra dei Greci, della quale poscia ambedue morirono; l'una *Teresa Portelli* il 1o. giugno 1851, ancòra di anni 19, e l'altra *Catterina*, l'epoca della cui morte non posso precisare, non avendola io curato fino agli ultimi periodi della malattia. Mi resta ora a notarle un fatto importante, massime perchè Ella, citando un autore moderno, dice "che la lebbra non sembra propagarsi per contagio, come la massima parte delle dermatosi squammose." *Carmela Portelli*, che era la domestica delle suddette *Portelli*, (colle quali non avea comune che il nome, non avendo avuto con esse nissuna parentela) pochi anni dopo loro morte, infermò della lebbra alla quale soccombette addì 10 decembre 1863, sotto cura del Sig. dott. Adami, che diagnosticò il caso a tempo per elefanziasi dei Greci. Se Ella crede che giovi per informazione dei lettori del suo periodico pubblicare questa notizia, V. S. è padrone di farlo. Intanto mi creda suo amico

Dott. Innocenzio Sammut.

3. T. Zammit. Malta and Mediterranean Branch. British Medical Journal, 1902 Jun 28; 1(2165): 1651–1656.

- Presents a case of leprosy treated with Dr. Carrasquilla's serum.

MALTA AND MEDITERRANEAN BRANCH.

A GENERAL meeting of this Branch was held on May 30th at Valetta under the presidency of Surgeon-General T. O'FARRELL, R.A.M.C. There were present twelve other members and visitors.

Confirmation of Minutes.—The minutes of the last meeting were read, confirmed, and signed.

Communications.—Dr. THEM. ZAMMIT read notes of a case of leprosy treated with Dr. Carrasquilla's serum.

The patient was about 32 when she came under his notice; she had been married fourteen years, and up to her seventh year of married life she enjoyed perfect health. At the seventh year of marriage she had her fourth child, and the first symptoms appeared when this child was 1 year old. The case was of the nodular variety, and when Dr. Zammit first saw her she had a typical leonine face, numerous nodosities on the arms and legs, and large patches of discoloration of the skin, and anaesthesia. The case was under the treatment of Dr. E. Meli of Valetta, who, having got a supply of the serum, asked Dr. Zammit if he was willing to make the injections. Dr. Zammit began the treatment at once, and injected eleven doses, about 10 c.cm. each, with an average interval of ten days. The injections were made with all antiseptic precautions, alternately at each side of the abdominal walls. No untoward effects were observed, no local action, nor skin eruption up to the eleventh injection. The patient became cheerful, and her aspect improved and lost its leonine character. After the eleventh injection the patient failed to make an appearance for about a month. When she came back she had a swollen red face; the nodosities all over the limbs were swollen to the size of a pigeon's egg, and the legs had the appearance of bags full of nuts. She said that the night after the last injection she had a long shiver, and felt hot and dizzy. She remained feverish for several days, with loss of appetite and general *malaise*, all the nodules on her body increasing in size. No pain or swelling was observed at the point of injection, and therefore an infection caused by the puncture of the syringe can be excluded. This strong reaction was not dissimilar to that observed after the injection of tuberculin in tuberculous patients, though Dr. Zammit could not understand why it occurred after the eleventh injection. About two months after this occurrence a marked improvement occurred. All the nodosities of the skin disappeared completely, and the dark patches and the anaesthetic areas faded away. The face assumed its normal aspect, and even the eyebrows covered themselves again with healthy hair. The improvement was so marked that he did not think of further injections. The woman, who had not borne children for the last six years, became pregnant again, and she gave birth to a fine healthy boy which she suckled. This pregnancy did not, however, improve the health of the mother, for when she was last seen, a few days before the date of the meeting, she had a few small nodules on the face and on one of the legs two ulcerations of a suspicious nature remained after a bruise she had sustained. The patient was most probably under the influence of the toxic products of Hansen's bacillus once more.

Dr. Zammit thought the case worth notice on account of the improvement following so markedly after the injections that it amounted almost to a cure. It should, he said, be borne in mind that the patient continued to lead the same old life amidst infected surroundings, with hard work and poor food. He believed that had she been treated in a sanatorium the improvement should have been permanent. He had seen many cases of leprosy treated with the ordinary drugs, but none had he seen improve so steadily as the case described.— A discussion followed in which Surgeon-General O'FARRELL, Lieutenant-Colonel SWABY, R.A.M.C., Major O'CONNOLL, R.A.M.C., Surgeon-Captain SAMUT, R.M.R., and Lieutenant KENNEDY, R.A.M.C., joined.—Dr. ZAMMIT then replied.

4. D. Spiteri, J. Guillaumier. Il-Lebbra: Il-kura nstabet iżda l-istigma għadha hemm? In-Nazzjon, 9th April 1994, p.17-19

Il-LEBBRA: Il-kura nstabet iżda l-istigma għadha hemm?

Minn Doris SPITERI, Ritratti John GUILLAUMIER

FORSI ftit huma dawk li jafu li fil-Għargħur jeżisti post magħruf bħala Ħal Ferħa. F'dan il-post hemm ħames residenti li ilhom hemm sa mit-13 ta' Diċembru ta' l-1974. Iżda għaliex u min huma dawn ir-residenti?

Il-ħames persuni residenti, żewġ nisa u tliet irġiel qabel ma sabu ruħhom Ħal Ferħa kien jinsabu f'sessjoni ta' l-isptar San Bartolomew (fejn illum jinsab Ħas-Serħ). Din is-sessjoni kienet riservata għall-pazjenti li kellhom il-lebbra. Dak iż-żmien jiġifieri fis-snin ta' wara it-tieni gwerra dinjija, il-marda tal-lebbra kienet mifruxa iżda mhux b'mod esaġerat.

Skond *warrant* li li kien inħareġ dak iż-żmien kull pazjent li jkun qed ibati minn din il-marda kellu jinġabar u b'hekk isib ruħu fi swali riservati apposta f'dan l-isptar. Din kienet prekawzjoni biex il-marda ma tibqax tinfirex.

Dan il-*warrant* tneħħa fl-1953 u għalhekk kienu bosta li reġgħu ngħaqdu mal-familjari tagħhom. Il-post li kienu jokkupaw fl-isptar San Bartolomew kien meħtieġ biex jilqa' aktar anzjani, għalhekk kien deċiz li dawk kollha li kienu baqgħu hemm jiġu trasferiti f'Ħal Ferħa. B'kollox kienu 23. Dawn kienu mqassma f'appartamenti individwali.

Maż-żmien kien hemm min telaq minn Ħal-Ferħa, kien hemm min sab impjieg u kien hemm min sab akkomodazzjoni alternattiva. Għal snin twal issa r-residenti ta' Ħal Ferħa niżlu għal ħames persuni.

Jibqa' fatt li mferrxa ma' Malta kollha hawn reġistrati madwar 80 persuna bil-marda tal-lebbra.

Din il-marda bla dubju ta' xejn iġġorr warajha ċerta stigma. Fl-1972, grazzi għal *Borstel Research Institute* tal-Ġermanja tal-Punent u għall-ħidma tal-professur Friskin il-pazjenti kollha tal-lebbra bdew ikunu mogħtija kura magħrufa bħala (MDT) *multiple drug therapy*.

Illum il-ġurnata ma teżistix klinika apposta fejn jiġu kkurati pazjenti lebrużi. Dan bi skop li titnaqqas l-istigma. Il-lebbra fiż-żmien ftit 'il bogħod kienet marda li tittieħed, iżda permezz tal-kura ġdida il-periklu illum spiċċa għal kollox.

Il-lebbra ilha taffettwa lill-bniedem aktar minn 2000 sena. Il-maġġoranza tagħhom jinsabu fil-pajjiżi anqas privileġġjati, l-aktar f'dawk tropikali.

Sfortunatament 30 fil-mija biss tal-morda bil-lebbra jistgħu jibbenefikaw mill-kura adattata.

Sadattant f'Malta kienu rappurtati tliet każijiet ġodda tal-lebbra fl-1989. L-ebda każ ma kien rappurtat fl-1990 u l-1991. L-aħħar każ ta' lebbra kien rappurtat fl-1992. Is-sena li għaddiet ma kien irrappurtat l-ebda każ.

Min huma r-residenti f'Tal-Ferħa Estate?

META dħalt f'Tal Ferħa Estate ma kontx naf eżattament dak li se nsib. Iżda issa nista' nikteb dwar dak li sibt. Il-post hu xi ftit diżabitat, f'nofs il-kampanja. Laqagħni Carmel Abela, l-Principal Nursing Officer li wara li tana informazzjoni dwar il-post laqqagħni mar-residenti.

Salvu, 66 sena

Iltqajt ma' Salvu forsi f'ġurnata ftit ħażina. Ftit tal-ħin qabel kien għadu kif mietlu l-ġeru ta' ħames xhur li kien qed irabbi. "Kien jiġdimni iżda kont inħobbu u nieħu ħsiebu. Minn meta abbandunawh wara l-bieb ta' l-Estate, ħadt grazzja miegħu u meta mort insaħħanlu ftit ħalib, ħatfu u bħal donnu għaraf li rridlu l-ġid"

Issa Salvu bħal speċi għamel f'qalbu iżda ma jridx irabbi kelb ieħor għaliex ma jridx li jkollu telfa oħra.

Madankollu Salvu xorta waħda rrakkuntali l-istorja tiegħu. "Jien kont inbiegħ is-saħħa, kont ħaddiem tat-tarzna u moħħ ir-riħ." Salvu jiftakar kif missieru kien miet minħabba li kellu l-lebbra.

Jum fost l-oħrajn mar għand it-Tabib Vincenti għaliex ma setax jieħu nifs minn imnieħru. "It-tabib qalli li kelli l-laħam ħażin. Kien bagħtni għand tabib ieħor, it-Tabib Azzopardi u meta dħalt għandu għamilli diversi eżamijiet u ċċekkjali l-urina. Wara li ħa d-dettalji tiegħi staqsieni missieri biex kien miet. Ksaħt u gdibt għax għidtlu li miet bil-kliewi. Qalli biex nerġa' mmur u nieħu miegħi lil ommi."

Salvu hekk għamel u ommu ħadet ix-xokk ta' ħajjitha meta t-tabib qalilha li binha marid bil-lebbra. Qalilna li minħabba l-liġi jrid ikun segregat biex ikun jista' jirċievi l-kura meħtieġa.

"Ommi bdiet tibki kemm tiflaħ u waqgħet ma l-art. Morna lura d-dar B'Kara b'tal-linja. Sibna lil ħija d-dar u għidnilu b'kollox." Huh bħal donnu nħasad. U min naħa tiegħu kien mar ukoll għand il-professur u tah l-istess aħbar kerha.

Dak iż-żmien qabel ma jinġabru fl-isptar San Batolomew, kienu jridu jgħaddu speċi ta' bord fl-isptar ċentrali (fejn illum jinsab il-Kwartieri tal-pulizija.). "Hija għalkemm seta' jiskapulaha ddeċieda li jinġabar miegħi u għalhekk ommi flok assistiet għal traġedja ta' wieħed ħadet ta' tnejn.

"Hemmhekk konna (jiġifieri jien u hija) inrabbu l-fniek u b'xi mod konna ngħadduha. Ftit taż-żmien wara mietet ommi. L-għali ma felħitx għalih."

Il-fatt li Salvu joqgħod Ħal-Ferħa ma jdejqu xejn. Hu jiftakar li meta kien spiċċa il-warrant hu kien ċarrat f'bosta biċċiet id-dokument tas-segregazzjoni.

Illum il-ġurnata Salvu jqatta' l-ġurnata jew jaħdem ir-raba inkella jpitter. Meta kien għadu żgħir kien imur l-iskola ta' l-arti għaliex il-pittura minn dejjem kienet tinteressah.

"Id-dar fadal biss oħti ż-żgħira. Ġieli mmur naraha għaliex għandi l-karrozza. Noħroġ nixtri wkoll għaliex jien ma nidhirx li kont marid. Naturalment naħbi l-identità tiegħi għaliex hemm nies li għadhom jibżgħu."

Waqt li kont qed nippassiġġa u nitħaddet ma' Salvu wasal tal-ħobż, għalhekk kelli nħallih ħalli jixtri bil-kwiet. Inkella ma kienx ikollu x'jiekol mal-aljotta li kien ippprepara għalih u għal ħuh.

Ara wkoll paġni 18 u 19

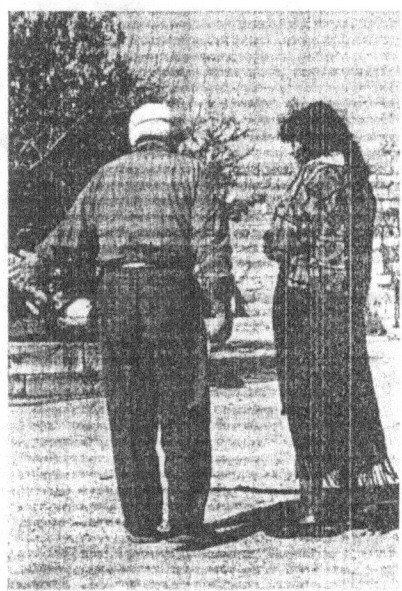

Salvu, resident f'Tal-Ferħa Estate, jitkellem ma' Doris SPITERI

Toni, 72 sena
Dejjem jitbissem minkejja t-tbatija

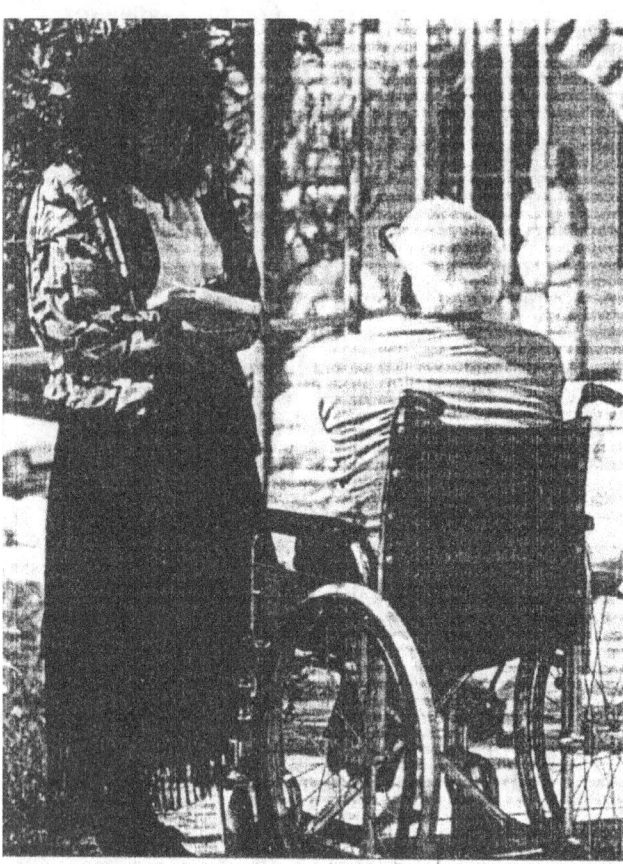

Toni: karattru ferrieħi minkejja s-sofferenzi kollha li għadda minnhom.

FTIT li xejn iltqajt ma' karattri allegri bħal dak ta' Toni. Minħabba kumplikazzjonijiet tad-diabete, Toni jinsab f' *wheelchair* għax qatgħulu sieq waħda.

Toni jgħid li ħuh Salvu jieħu ħafna ħsiebu u mn'alla kien hu għalih. Toni wkoll għandu storja x'jirrakkonta....

"Meta jien u ħija skoprejna dak li mradna bih, bħal speċi eċitajna ruħna u ma konniex nafu eżattament x'se naqbdu nagħmlu. Kien hemm tabib li ssuġġerili li mmur Tunis għaliex hemm ma kien hemm l-ebda *warrant*. Jien ma xtaqtx ninfired mill-familja u għalhekk għażilt li nibqa' ma' ħija".

Toni għadu jiftakar iż-żmien taż-żgħożija meta kien joħroġ mal-ġuvintur u tfajliet u ta' spiss kien imur ir-Rocky Vale. Minn fuq il-gazzetta kien ikun jaf b'kull *dance* li jkun organizzat. Kien fuq tiegħu u dak iż-żmien kellu namrata li kienet infermiera fl-Isptar Ċentrali.

"Kont qed inħoss uġigħ fl-għadam. Ix-xogħol tiegħi kien fuq il-ktajjen id-*dockyard* għalhekk kont inbati ħafna. Kienet proprju n-namrata li għamlitli appuntament mal-professur. Tani l-aħbar ħażina u fl-isptar flok mort waħdi mort jien u hija"

Toni jgħid li hu u ħuh għarfu jadattaw ruħhom. "Hija jgħini ħafna u nista' ngħid li salvali ħajti. Għall-bidu tajtha għax-xorb. Kont nesaġera iżda ħija kien bil-għaqal u kien dejjem jipprova jiftaħli għajnejja. Il-bniedem ma tridx tiġġudikah mid-daħka ta' fuq fommu. Wieħed irid iħares 'il ġewwa, fil-fond fejn jinsabu l-vera feriti.

"Meta kien ikolli ftit tal-kumpannija kont inġagħħa iżda malli kont insib ruħi waħdi kont indur lejn sieħbi x-xorb. Kont inpejjep ħafna wkoll u rnexxili naqtagħhom biss, sentejn ilu."

Toni sofra mhux ħażin iżda xorta waħda rnexxilu jżomm tbissima fuq fommu. Karattru ferrieħi li ma tantx għadek issib fil-ħajja mgħaġġla ta' kuljum.

Marija, 70 sena
'M'għandix għalfejn nistħi u għalfejn ninħeba'

MARIJA laqgħetni fl-appartament ċkejken tagħha daqs li kieku kont waħda tal-familja. Mara simpatika u fuq tagħha mhux ħażin, iżda kuxjenzjuża u ġeneruża għall-aħħar.

Marija tirrakkonta li ħadet il-marda meta kellha biss 17-il sena. Kienet tfajla mill-isbaħ iżda meta waslet biex issir xebba bdiet tħoss l-ewwel sintomi u minn xahar għall-ieħor baqgħet sejra lura.

"Il-marda qatt ma ħadtha bis-serjetà, kont tip li naf inderri u bqajt attiva, kont inħobb ninnittja iżda meta bdejt nitlef l-użu ta' jdejja ma stajtx inkompli. Din kienet l-aktar ħaġa li tefgħetni lura. Ma' tal-familja mhux possibli li ngħix għaliex ma ridtx inkun ta' piż. Waħdi lanqas stajt ngħix għaliex ma stajtx inkun autosuffiċjenti.

"Meta ġabruni San Bartolomew ma kontx kuntenta għaliex hemm konna fi swali u ma kellniex spazju għalina. Meta qaluli li se jeħduna post ieħor ma kontx naf x'se nsib, iżda meta sibt li se jkolli dari u fl-istess waqt xorta kien se jkolli għajnuna, ħassejtni kuntenta ħafna.

"Dan l-aħħar il-ġurnata inqattagħha quddiem it-televiżjoni. Ma nfallix episodju wieħed tar-rumanzi u tat-telenovelas. Insegwihom minn filgħodu sa meta jispiċċaw. Dawn il-programmi saru ħajti.

"Jien la jien ħabsija u lanqas qatt m'għamilt xejn ħażin. Il-marda ma ġibthiex fuqi għax ridt jien u għalhekk la għandi għalfejn nistħi u lanqas għalfejn ninħeba. Hawnhekk ninsab kuntenta u kulma nitlob hu li jħalluni hawn għall-kwiet."

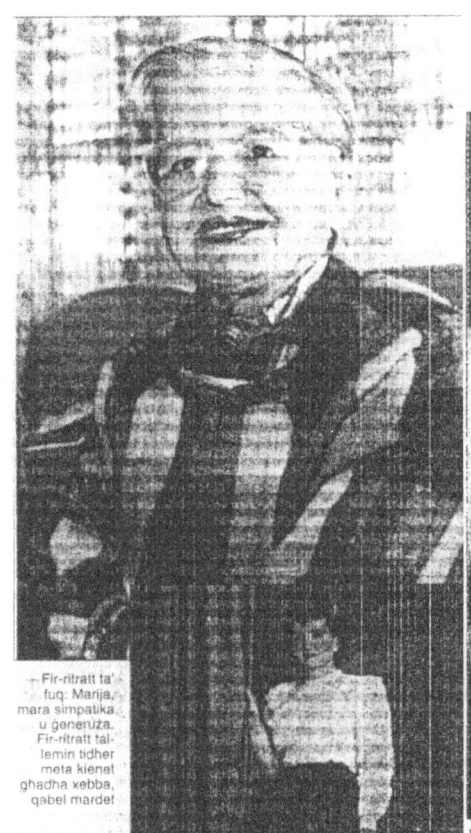
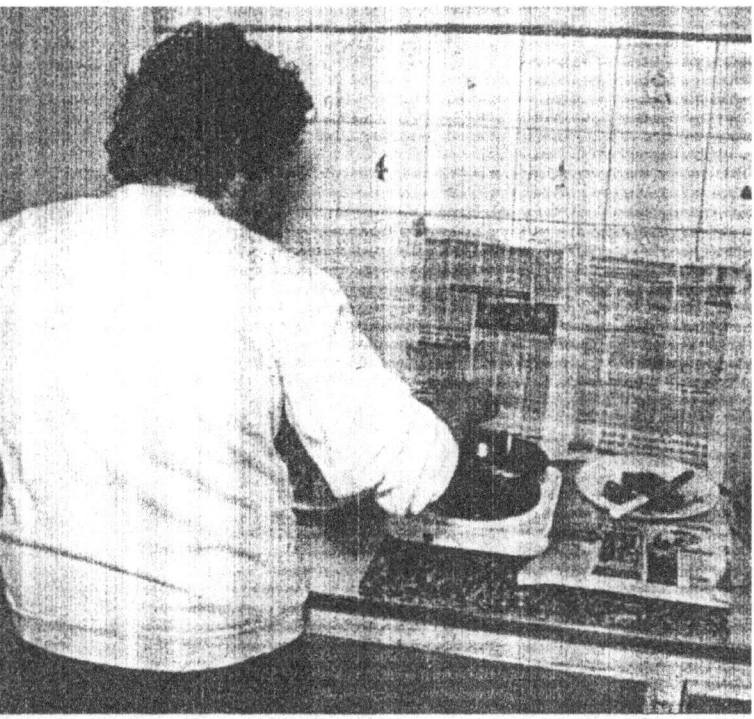

Fir-ritratt ta' fuq: Marija, mara simpatika u ġeneruża. Fir-ritratt tal-lemin tidher meta kienet għadha xebba, qabel mardet

Vitor: il-gost tagħha fil-kċina

Vitor, 68 sena
'Iż-żminijiet koroh għaddew'

LIL Vitor dħalt niddisturbaha fil-kċina waqt li kienet qed taqli l-ħut. Sinċerament ir-riħa li bdiet ħierġa qabbditni ġuħ kbir.

Vitor ukoll kienet mardet meta kienet għadha daqsxejn ta' tfajla. Kellha eżattament 17-il sena. Hi tgħid li għaddiet minn żminijiet koroh iżda llum tgħid li dak iż-żmien għadda. Ma' tal-familja għandha kuntatt tajjeb u ta' sikwit tmur tarahom. Ommha u missierha m'ilhomx wisq li mietu iżda hi kellha l-opportunità li ddur bihom.

"In-nies daż-żmien ma tantx għadhom jagħtu kas. Jiġi minni jekk noqgħod lura. Hawnekk jiġu bosta żgħażagħ u gruppi u jorganizzawlna bar-b-ques u attivitajiet oħra. Naturalment jkolli mumenti ta' solitudini iżda dejjem insib f'hiex nehda, t-tisjir u l-faċendi jokkupali bosta ħin."

Lil Vitor ħallejtha mattagen u l-ħut filwaqt li fuq l-għatba tal-bieb bdiet riesqa daqsxejn ta' qattusa li għal dan l-aħħar żmien iddabbar xi ħaġa x'tiekol mingħand Vitor.

Ħajja ta' kuraġġ u determinazzjoni

MILL-ĦAMES residenti ta' Ħal-Ferħa, Grezzju ma setax jagħtini l-kummenti tiegħu għaliex kien barra bil-karrozza. Sħabu r-residenti l-oħra jgħidu li Grezzju hu pjuttost raġel attiv u ma jaqta' qalbu minn xejn.

Maria, Vitor, Salvu u Toni qasmu flimkien l-istess destin għal aktar minn erbgħin sena. Għexu flimkien ħajja ta' rassenjazzjoni iżda b'kuraġġ u determinazzjoni kbira.

Minkejja kollox għarfu japprezzaw il-ħajja, jafu jitbissmu u jeħdew fil-passatempi tagħhom. Irnexxielhom jirbħu l-kruha tas-solitudini.

Kulma baqa' issa hu li s-soċjetà kollha jirnexxilha tirbaħ għal kollox l-istigma inutili li kultant għadha żżomm f'qalbha għal dawn in-nies.

Kura kontra l-lebbra nstabet. Li jonqos hu li jitfejjaq min għadu indifferenti u għadu ma rebaħx l-istigma bla sens fil-konfront ta' persuni b'din il-marda.

5. T.A. Reed: Leprosy beyond the year 2000. *Lancet*, 1998, 351(9104):p.757.

"Sir, Anecdote may carry little weight in these days of meta-analysis, but in view of statements in your Dec 13 editorial, I will relate the history of the first case of leprosy seen and treated by me in the Spring of 1944 in Malta where I was a trainee dermatovenereologist in the Royal Army Medical Corps.

He was a previously healthy, UK born, gunner aged 22, who had arrived on the island in 1941, became friendly with a Maltese girl in 1942, and visited her home to take tea, at infrequent intervals (rationing 1500 cals daily did not permit more lavish hospitality). In 1942, the leper hospital close to RAF Luqa Aerodrome was bombed, and the patients sent to their homes, including the girl's father who had lepromatous leprosy. She was clinically and microscopically negative for the leprosy bacillus, and the only indirect contact was via the house tea cups. Due to shortages of fuel and detergents, the washing-up can best be described as perfunctory. The gunner first noticed puffiness of his face in the autumn of 1943, some 18 months after his first visit to take tea.

The failure of the perfunctory washing-up to cleanse fomites was also illustrated by the fact that hepatitis A was ten times more common in officers and sergeants whose cutlery and crockery was washed together and shared, than amongst the other ranks who kept and cleaned their own. May I suggest that with modern PCR techniques the presence of B leprae on fomites could be confirmed."

C: Government Commissioned Reports

1. Report on Leprosy by the Royal College of Physicians prepared for Her Majesty's Secretary of State for the Colonies, with an Appendix. London, 1867. *Il Barth*, 6th August 1874, 3(21-22):424-427

Report on Leprosy by the Royal College of Physicians prepared for Her Majesty's Secretary of State for the Colonies, with an Appendix. London 1867.— Rapporto sulla Lebbra pel Collegio Reale dei Medici di Londra.

Un volume in foglio di 310 pagine includenti il rapporto la corrispondenza ed un'appendice. *(Sunto)*.

Ringraziamo di cuore l'onor. Sir Victor Houlton, Principale Segretario di Governo, di una copia del suddetto lavoro. Quantunque un po' fuori di data, avendo veduto la luce sette anni ora sono, pure non essendo stato tradotto in italiano e fornendo esso i materiali più ricchi per una compiuta monografia sulla elefantiasi dei Greci, non sarà forse fuori di luogo farlo conoscere ai nostri lettori con un breve sunto e valendoci delle varie contribuzioni pubblicate nei giornali medici, su questo argomento, terremo conto dei soccorsi terapeutici che, insin dalla pubblicazione del rapporto, vennero consigliati in questa ribelle affezione.

La lebbra si manifesta colle medesime note caratteristiche in tutte le regioni dov'essa esercita il suo triste impero. Un'eruzione cutanea, gravi disordini del processo nutritivo, tendenza alla ulcerazione ed alla necrosi delle parti colpite, disturbi dell'innervazione, debolezza o totale mancanza della sensibilità; ecco le note caratteristiche di cotesta formidabile egritudine. Le due forme, già ammesse in sin da remoto tempo dagli scrittori, di questa infermità, sembrano veramente distinte, e sono (1) la *tubercolosa*, o meglio *tubercolata*, perchè l'epiteto non possa destare alcuna idea della tubercolosi, morbo affatto distinto; (2) l'*anestetica*, la quale, alla sua volta, conviene meglio designare col nome di *non-tubercolata*, conciossiacchè nella tubercolata avverinsi spesso dei punti anestetici. Come sotto varietà della non-tubercolata hassi da riguardare *la lebbra leucopatica*, di cui abbiamo dato la descrizione in una delle precedenti dispense colla storia di un caso; in questa le chiazze anche presentano i fenomeni di difettosa innervazione.

Non crediamo utile dare qui un'ampia descrizione della lebbra, imperochè con dipintura raffaellesca ce ne trasmisero i caratteri gli autori del medio-evo; ed è provato colla più chiara evidenza che la elefantiasi dei Greci si presenta oggigiorno colla stessa fenomenologia, come nei secoli di mezzo, il che anche si inferisce da una descrizione del morbo, la quale il dott. Wilson aggiunse al rapporto di cui andiam facendo il riassunto.

La lebbra è un morbo di tutte le età: gli stessi neonati dei lebbrosi offrono talvolta segni di questa degenerazione. Fu erroneo adunque quanto insegnava il Billard la elefantiasi dei Greci non essere stata mai osservata nella prima infanzia.

Alla comparsa dei segni caratteristici della lebbra spesso succede il seguente treno sintomatico: malessere generale, rigori di freddo, febbriciattola, dolori e formicolio negli arti, ottusa sensibilità in una mano o in un piede o in un dito, mancanza di vigore fisico e morale, e, secondo Jackson e Martin, un abbondante sudore dalle mani, che n'è riguardato come uno dei caratteri della diatesi lebbrosa. Ei sembra che il decorso della malattia non sia lo stesso nelle sue due forme, imperochè è stato notato la lebbra non-tubercolata essere di lunga mano più lenta della tubercolata, e un arresto del progresso del morbo verificarsi più presto nella non-tubercolata, anzichè nell'altra. Ordinariamente la vita del lebbroso è spenta da un morbo intercorrente, come sarebbe a dire da diarrea, dissenteria, bronchite e polmonite. La malaria esercita sul lebbroso un'influenza assai malefica, infatti un solo attacco di febbre intermittente o remittente, detta febbre biliosa dei paesi caldi, basta assai sovente per troncargli la misera esistenza. Anche le malattie renali, non rare fra i lebbrosi, per lo più tornano loro esiziali. Fra le degenerazioni più comuni quella conosciuta sotto il nome di morbo brightico cronico è la più frequente ed assieme la più fatale. La lebbra sembra prescegliere di frequenza i maschi, i popoli di pelle oscura e nera, le genti basse e povere, quantunque essa risparmi le civili e le ricche. Questa terribile infermità esercita maggior strage nelle regioni basse e maremmose, nei paesi marittimi e nelle città. Molti asseverano, non sappiamo con quanta ragione, che l'uso costante del pesce salato, stantio o semiputrido favorisce lo sviluppo della lebbra più di qualunque altro alimento: così anche l'olio rancido, e certi legumi: vuolsi anche che la mancanza di carne fresca e di vegetabili la favorisca d'assai.

I medici tutti sono unanimi nell'annoverare fra le cause della degenerazione in parola: la dieta malsana ed inefficiente, le vicissitudini atmosferiche, le case umide e sporche, la mancanza di nettezza della persona, l'intemperanza, la venere smodata, e tutto ciò che può determinare l'aglobulia, come sono le preparazioni mercuriali. Che la lebbra sia un'infermità ereditaria non è da dubitare; continue osservazioni confermano cosiffatta verità: ciò non ostante essa sviluppasi eziandio in persone che non vi sortirono dalla nascita nessuna tendenza. È ora mai noto che i lebbrosi ponno generare figli sceveri della benchè minima traccia di questa spaventevole lue: non di rado in alcuni non se ne manifesta di là di un'adenite cervicale, accompagnata o no da un colorito spanemico; altri offrono segni di viziosa conformazione, o sono rachitici, oppure astenici, e in molti di essi lo sviluppo dell'organismo s'arresta in modo che fatti maturi sembrano tuttavia fanciulli cachettici o sono tisicuzzi nani.

Egli è necessario che il pratico sappia come nei figli dei lebbrosi, le comuni infermità, quelle appunto che in altri bambini riescono facilmente curabili, sieno per lo più ribelli e spessissimo anche mortali; dal che si inferisce quanto sia piccola la resistenza organica a questi infelici trasmessa dai parenti. Come avviene nella tisa, nella gotta e in altri morbi ereditarii, anche nella elefantiasi dei Greci s'avverano i maravigliosi e non ancora ben spiegati esempi di atavismo. Ritengono i medici cinesi, come anche gli europei, che esercitano la medicina nella Cina, che la degenerazione lebbrosa perde di forza passando attraverso vari organismi, e che dopo un tempo finisce per esaurirsi del tutto; e recano prove numerose e ad un tempo ineluttabili, che nella terza generazione i fenomeni morbosi cessano di essere così terribili come si erano manifesi nella prima e nella seconda, e che nella quarta se la lue non è compiutamente estinta, essa è per lo meno benigna.

Pensarono alcuni che le due forme summenzionate della lebbra dei Greci avessero due distinti origini, e fossero anzi due entità patologiche separate: ma quanto fossero costoro lontani dalla esattezza desumesi dal fatto che un lebbroso spesso trasmette ad un figlio l'una, e ad un altro l'altra delle due forme: oltre a ciò non sono rari gli esempi di egri in cui le forme tubercolata, e non-tubercolata s'osservano insieme combinate.

Pretesero diversi patologi che la lebbra fosse originata dalla sifilide, la quale Proteo delle malattie d'infezione, ha una forma tubercolata che ben rassomiglia la degenerazione lebbrosa: ma quanto sia poco sostenibile cotesta origine si inferisce dal fatto che in Nuova Brunswick e nel nord della Persia, la sifilide è ignota, mentre la lebbra vi regna endemica.

Nei casi piuttosto frequenti in cui il paziente è imbrattato dalla lue sifilitica riesce sommamente difficile il conoscere la vera natura dell'affezione.

In alcuni casi, è vero, non si può non confondere colla lebbra la framboesia, detta *yaws* dagli Americani (micosi dell'Alibert): ma quei che ritengono queste due infermità avere la stessa origine anzi la stessa natura, l'errano di lunga mano, poichè mentre la elefantiasi è cosmopolita; la framboesia, altre volte frequentissima nelle Isole dell'India occidentale, è una dermopatia contagiosa, oggidì piuttosto rara e confinata in certe regioni. Evvi uno stato morboso, non menzionato nel Rapporto, il quale potendosi confondere colla lebbra dei Greci, è mestieri che i pratici ne sieno avvertiti; quest'è l'*artrite deformante*, abbastanza frequente da noi, e non di rado complicata con dermopatie squammose, massime la psoriasi, affezione astenica che attacca di frequenza individui di debole costituzione e già acciaccati da croniche infermità. Le autorità più rispettabili sembrano convenire la lebbra non essere contagiosa, nè trasmissibile per congressi sessuali: anche Von Someren, citato in un'altra pagina di questa dispensa, sostiene cotesta dottrina.

Quanto al trattamento i medici più sperimentati sono unanimi nel considerare l'igiene come l'unica risorsa per ritardare ed arrestare il progresso dell'egritudine nei suoi primi stadi e per mitigarne la severità quando ben sviluppata. Nella già menzionata contribuzione del Wilson, questo insigne erpetologo considerando che tale morbo esprime una pessima assimilazione, assennatamente insegna che nessun soccorso vi può avere alcuna efficacia, il quale non valga a rielevare il processo nutritivo. La comune dei medici ritiene che nissun modificatore farmaceutico esercita un'azione favorevole su questo terribile morbo: imperocchè, è uopo pur confessarlo, l'olio di *Chaulmoogra odorata*, la *Calotropis gigantea*, ed altre sostanze vegetabili, alle quali un cieco empirismo ad una pratica poco illuminata avevano attribuito qualità curative nella lebbra, non vi esercitano nissuna benefica influenza. Ed i vari soccorsi farmaceutici stati impiegati da sette anni a questa parte, vogliam dire dalla pubblicazione del rapporto in esame, sono oggigiorno generalmente abbandonati, siccome avvertiva, testè il dott. Gavin Milroy, appoggiandosi ai risultati ottenuti da Von Someren nel Madras, e da Poupinel° de Valence nell'Isola Borbone, i quali sono amendue convinti che l'olio di *Anacardium occidentale* (*Oil of cashew-nut*) da loro impiegato su larga scala e preconizzato da molti con grande entusiasmo nella lebbra, non è valevole a combattere cotesta formidabile malattia.

È stato testè annunziato come prezioso agente curativo l'*olio o balsamo di gurgiun*, detto *Wood oil*, olio di legno, dagli Indiani, che insin da lungo tempo lo lodano per i suoi pronti effetti nella blenorragia. Esso è un essudato oleo-resinoso di varie specie della famiglia delle *Dipterocarpee*. Il dott. Dougall lo adoperò esternamente ed internamente in vari casi di lebbra, e ne ottenne effetti vantaggiosi, come asserisce egli nel lavoro che ha per titolo: *Report on the Treatment of Leprosy with Gurjun oil* by J. Dougall M.D. *Calcutta* 1874. A tale lavoro faceva eco non ha guari il dott. Dyce Duckworth, attestante il beneficio attenuto da un lebbroso ricoverato nello Ospedale di San Bartolomeo di Londra, dal doppio uso esterno ed interno del balsamo di Gurgiun. Questi fatti che non sono bastevoli per alcuna conchiusione, devono certamente invogliare il pratico a nuove esperienze.

Intorno al mercurio stesso l'esperienza si è maggiormente dichiarata, come si evince dalle seguenti parole del De Valencé: "*Cette medication n' à rien produit sur nos malades, et son action trop prolongée aurait fini par leur être nuisible*". Egli è dalla buon aria, dai buoni alimenti, dall'idroterapia in unione ai tonici ferruginosi e vegetabili, che devesi aspettare qualche miglioramento. Dalle preparazioni arsenicali adoperate da molti pratici non sembra che si sia ottenuto niuusn vantaggio reale.

La lebbra non guarisce spontaneamente; ed allorchè è sviluppata con tutte le sue note caratteristiche la materia medica non possiede soccorsi atti a debellarla: essa allora è incurabile! È vero che il progresso se ne può ritardare ed anche per un tempo arrestare, quando il paziente è in favorevoli condizioni igieniche; pure la terminazione è costantemente la morte o per marasmo o per un qualsiasi morbo intercorrente: e la morte spesso s'invoca dal lebbroso confermato,

......" A cui il morire
Più amaro sarà, quanto più tardo".

Ai dott. Danielssen e Boeck, che hanno dissettato molti cadaveri di lebbrosi, dobbiamo le nostre attuali conoscenze sui cambiamenti morbosi, che han luogo in cotesti infermi: eglino riscontrarono nella forma tubercolata; ingrossamento della mucosa faringo-laringea, depositi morbosi nella laringe, tubercoli nella mucosa bronco-tracheale, adeniti cervicali, ingrossamento delle pleure, ingrossamento delle glandole mesenteriche, ulcerazioni intestinali, degenerazioni renali, massime quelle che sono proprie della nefrite albuminosa cronica: e nella non-tubercolata, detta anestetica; atrofie muscolari, ingrossamento dei nervi, che traversano i tessuti offesi dalla lue, ingorghi ascellari ed inguinali e vari cambiamenti patologici nel sistema nervoso centrale.

È stato già detto che la lebbra affligge l'umanità in tutte le regioni: nè senza ragione i chiarissimi estensori della relazione in parola misero in dubbio l'asserzione di parecchi medici i quali, appoggiati alla propria esperienza, ritennero la lebbra non svilupparsi in certi paesi; esempligrazia, Nuova Scozia, Malta, le Isole Malnine, Sant'Elena, Trebisonda, Natal, Gibilterra ecc: Che in Malta di quando in quando si osservi questa schifosa egritudine l'abbiam già dimostrato? (pag.) e gli autori della relazione citano Danielssen e Boeck, i quali considerano quest'isola come una delle sedi della lebbra: ed a calce del testo riproducono le parole del dott. Fowler, che narra come persone tuttora viventi in Sant'Elena rammentino avervi osservato infermi di elefantiasi, la quale per altro da poco tempo non più vi si manifesta, forse per migliorate condizioni igieniche di quell'isola.

Quanto alla distribuzione geografica della lebbra crediamo che pochi fatti siano stati aggiunti dai medici del Collegio Reale a quelli già prima conosciuti: ed in vero eglino stimarono prezzo della opera (pag. 227) l'esibire un sunto dell'opera classica di Hirsch intitolata *Handbuch der Historisch — geographschen Pathologie*.

2. Contagiosita` della elefantiasi dei Greci. *Il Barth : gazzetta di medicina e scienze naturali*, 6 August 1874, 3(21-22):442

> **Contagiosità della elefantiasi dei Greci.**
> Il dott. W. J. Van Someren in una lettera che egli indirige dal Madras al *Medical Times and Gazette*, in risposta ad un articolo comparso nel *British and Foreign Medico-chirurgical Review*, intorno alla trasmissibilità della elefantiasi greca per via di contagio, il celebre erpetologo nega recisamente che tale morbo possa comunicarsi per contagio, per congressi sessuali, tampoco per inoculazione del sangue e delle materie saniose dei lebbrosi.

3. *Reports on Leprosy in Malta by a Committee appointed by H.E. the Governor in 1917. Final Report.* Government Printing Office, Malta, 1919

D: Leprosaria Reports – St. Bartholomew's Hospital, Malta and Sacred Heart Hospital, Gozo

1. Office of Charitable Institutions: *Reports on the Workings of Government Departments during the financial years 1900-1936.* Government Printing Office, Malta, 1901-1937, annual reports

2. Department of Health: *Annual Reports on the Health Conditions of the Maltese Islands and on the work of the Medical and Health Department for the years 1937-1971.* Department of Health, Malta, 1938-1972, annual reports.

    - Contain annual reports and statistics pertaining to the management of the various leprosaria and on the public health issues related to Hansen's disease.

3. Commons Sitting of 14 April 1943 Series 5 Vol. 388 - MALTA (MENTAL ASYLUM AND LEPER HOSPITAL). HC Deb 14 April 1943 vol 388 cc1231-2W1231W. *Commons and Lords Hansard, the Official Report of debates in Parliament.* https://api.parliament.uk/historic-hansard/written-answers/1943/apr/14/malta-mental-asylum-and-leper-hospital

    - Dr. Morgan asked the Secretary of State for the Colonies whether he is aware that in the island of Gozo, in the Crown Colony of Malta, the mental hospital, asylum, and the leper colony are in the same enclosure of an old walled building, inadequately separated by a wall and that one medical officer in charge acts as medical superintendent of both institutions; whether he will improve these arrangements; and what recent improvements have taken place in the dietaries of these places?
    - Colonel Stanley – The mental asylum and the leper hospital are within the same enclosing wall but are in separate buildings adequately separated by open grounds and an inner wall. Each institution is entirely self-contained. One resident medical superintendent is in charge of both institutions but the asylum is visited regularly by the medical superintendent of the mental hospital, Malta, and the leper colony is similarly visited by the leprosy control officer. The present arrangements are reported to be satisfactory. Since November, 1942, the dietary has been increased and improved in relation to

increases and improvements which I am very glad to say it has been possible to make in the dietary of the general population following a very material improvement in the supply position.

4. L. Farrer-Brown, H. Boldero, J.B. Oldham: *Report of the Medical Services Commission*. Central Office of Information, Malta, 1957, p.24
    - Describes the building and management of St. Bartholomew Hospital
    - Reports the closure of the Sacred Heart Hospital in Gozo.
        "St. Bartholomew Hospital: 95. Until recently there have been two hospitals for leper – St. Bartholomew Hospital in Malta and the Sacred Heart Hospital in Gozo. The Sacred Heart Hospital, which is at Fort Chambray alongside the Mental Hospital, had a bed compliment of 27 beds but was closed down in December last owing to lack of patients. 96. In Malta. As in Gozo, the number of lepers is steadily diminishing. St. Bartholomew Hospital, which is contiguous with St. Vincent de Paul Hospital, is an old but fine and spacious building. Its bed complement is 118 beds and at the present there are only 40 in-patients, as compared with an average of 75 patients in 1953 and 73 in 1954. There is one medical officer – the Medical Superintendent – but he is able to have regular off duty, one of the doctors from St. Vincent de Paul Hospital acting in his relief. St. Bartholomew Hospital has better amenities than many of the hospitals in Malta. The wards, the corridors and the gardens are spacious and pleasing. There is an entertainment hall and efforts are made to organize shows and outings for the patients. There is, however, room for improvement in the amenities and for help from voluntary workers."

5. A Healthy People – A Happy People. Ministry of Health, Malta, 1981, p.10-11
    - Records the change in services offered by St. Bartholomew Hospital from a leprosarium to an old people's hospice and the change of name to Ruzar Briffa Complex.
        "Has-Serh: St Bartholomew's Hospital, which was once reserved for leprous patients, and is located within the general complex of Has-Serh, was also modernized. Named after one of Malta's main writers, Ruzar Briffa, this hospital now offers more space within the complex for elderly citizens."

F: Folklore

1. G. Despott: The Reptiles of the Maltese Islands. *The Zoologist*, 15 September 1915, ser.IV, 19(891):321-326 (322).
    - Describes the Maltese folklore belief that geckos transmitted leprosy.
        "It is a common belief here that both our Geckos have the power of inflicting leprosy on those who touch them ; this is, however, only a prejudice, the poor creatures being perfectly harmless. This belief, however, is the cause of a most cruel persecution of these reptiles ; and so general is it also that, no matter how much good the offer one makes, he will find the greatest difficulty in getting a boy to collect Geckos for him."

G: Overall Reviews

6. J. Bugeja: Leprosy in Malta. *Reports on the working of Government departments during the financial year 1930-31.* Government Printing Office, Malta, 1932, R:p.17-30

Appendix A. R 17

LEPROSY IN MALTA.

Paper read by Dr. J. Bugeja, Junior Resident Assistant Superintendent and Medical Officer of the Poor House and of the Hospital for Lepers, at the School of Tropical Medicine at Calcutta.

The origin of leprosy in Malta is unknown. So far it has been usually held that, were it possible to trace back the first existence of the disease in the Island, one would probably find that it affected the earliest of its inhabitants. The situation of the Maltese Islands—180 miles off the Northern Coast of Africa, the excellent shelter afforded by their harbours to seafaring vessels from the Eastern Mediterranean, and the immigration from the surrounding leprosy-infected countries, are put forward as reasons which support this hypothesis.

It is more probable, however, that the first cases of leprosy were introduced into Malta through the influx of leprosy-infected Arabs, from the Eastern and Southern littorals of the Mediterranean during the Saracen domination between 870 and 1090 A.D. After the decline of the Byzantine Empire, the power of Islam spread rapidly westwards from Syria to Egypt and Carthage, the tribes overrunning these countries, subsequently invading Malta through Sicily. In support of this contention is the fact that the only Maltese word meaning leprosy is "djem" or "gdim", the origin of which is from "djudsam", the Arabic word for leprosy.

The exact history of leprosy in Malta is obscure before 1880. As a matter of fact the disease was completely ignored up to 1687, in which year five cases were recorded by Dr. Joseph Zammit, Professor of Medicine in the Medical School of the Order of St. John of Jerusalem. A further case was described by Dr. Saydon in 1808 and two other cases by Dr. Gravagna in 1837. It is also found that several references to leprosy were made in the debates held by a Maltese Medical Society which was in existence up to 1837.

It must not be assumed that, besides these authentic cases of leprosy, there were no others which went by unrecorded; but these latter must have been very few, and consequently the disease did not attract the attention of either the Medical Faculty or the Authorities. A gradual and steady increase, however, in the number of leprosy cases began to cause anxiety amongst the inhabitants in the year 1880, and in 1883 a Committee composed of seven medical practitioners was appointed by the Governor "to investigate and study the incidence of the disease and to suggest means to check its spread".

Four events, occurring during the twenty years immediately preceding 1883, have been important factors in increasing the incidence of leprosy in the Islands. Firstly, the cholera epidemics in 1865 and 1867; this disease, which may have prepared the soil for leprosy, was introduced from Egypt in the first case and by refugees from Tunisia in the second, both countries where leprosy is prevalent. Secondly, the opening of the Suez Canal in 1869: the mapping of a new route to the East greatly facilitated commercial intercourse between Malta and those countries where leprosy is also rife. Thirdly, the return of emigrants from the Northern Coast of Africa; for the first time in 1865 and again in 1872, owing to economic depression in Malta, batches of emigrants left the Island, and these would not proceed further than North Africa. The return of these emigrants was naturally a means of propagating the disease. Fourthly, the arrival in Malta in 1878, of a strong contingent of Indian troops; in connection with the Russo-Turkish War, Indian troops, numbering over 6000 men in all, were brought to Malta. This event was probably the most important cause of the increase of leprosy in the Islands, for these troops were stationed at Imriehel, a place situated in the position of a hub to those villages (Zebbug, Curmi, Birchircara, Naxaro), in which, according to the earliest statistics, leprosy cases were most numerous.

The main result of the labours of the Committee appointed in 1883, and the most important step ever taken so far in connection with leprosy, was the decision to segregate all leprosy-infected persons. Although the specific bacillus was discovered in 1873, heredity was in those days the dominant theory put forward to account for the transmission of leprosy; medical men in the Island maintained that view, although contagion was not excluded. Among the population, however, there was, and there is still, an exaggerated, if mistaken, apprehension of the contagiousness of leprosy. Segregation was the policy then generally adopted in most countries, especially in Europe. The local conditions of the Maltese Islands, with their restricted area of 121 square miles, and the small number of lepers, rendered compulsory segregation an ideal means for extinguishing the dread scourge.

Before recommending the segregation of lepers, the Committee had contemplated other methods for combating the disease, but each had to be discarded. Thus, for instance, isolation at the patients' own home, under the control of the Sanitary Authorities, was impracticable in view of the restricted financial means of the patients, who are drawn mostly from the poorer classes. The project of instituting a leper settlement on Comino, a small uninhabited Island between Malta and Gozo, had to be abandoned, because the number of lepers was not sufficiently large to warrant this scheme; also in view of the inadequate and difficult means of reaching this small Island from the mainland, especially in winter.

It will thus be observed that nothing was left undone by the local Government before the issue of the 1893 Lepers Ordinance entitled "An Ordinance for checking the spread of the disease commonly known as Leprosy", that is, ten years after the disease had first caused a stir among the people. The Ordinance was based on three predominant factors, namely:

i) Compulsory notification of every case of leprosy immediately it is recognized by medical men and by certain laymen, namely, Police Officers and persons holding the management of a lodging-house, hotel, etc., under pain of legal penalties for omission.

ii) Examination of each notified case by a Board of five experienced medical men, specially appointed, (styled the Leprosy Board).

iii) Segregation of confirmed leprosy cases in a Leprosarium so long as such cases are deemed to be a danger to the public.

The next problem facing the Government, a corollary to the Ordinance, was the erection of a suitable hospital for the isolation of lepers. Obviously, the main provision of the law of 1893 could not become operative, unless and until a special Institution was built. A small number of lepers, in an advanced stage of the disease, had of their own accord applied for admission into an Institution. These were isolated, as far as was practicable, in a ward of the Asylum for the Aged and Incurables, commonly known as the Poor House. A few years after the promulgation of the Lepers Ordinance, the erection of the Leper Asylum, known since 1919 as the Leper Hospital, was commenced at Imghieret, a solitary, somewhat elevated spot on the South-eastern side of the Island, three miles away from Valletta and about 200 yards from the Poor House, from which it is entirely separated.

**

With the beginning of the present century, the history of leprosy in Malta enters upon a new and a better authenticated phase. In 1900 one division of the Leprosarium was completed for the reception of male lepers. Since then, accurate statistics have been kept. The female division, however, was not opened until 1912, the great lapse of time between the erection of the two divisions being due to other commitments on the part of the Government. Thus, it was only in 1912 that compulsory segregation was made general, and whilst accurate records for male lepers can be obtained since the year 1900, statistics for female lepers are not available before 1912.

The Leper Hospital, as existing at the present day, is constructed on a plan of two lateral wings emerging at right angles from each side of a central block through long open corridors. The right wing is the male division, the left, the female section, while the central block is used as Offices for the administration. The main entrance, the vestibule and the chapel form part of this block. On either side of the vestibule are the residential quarters of the Sisters of Charity and of the Chaplain, the dispensary and stores. Beyond the chapel are the kitchen and the laundry. The two wings consist of wards accommodating from four to twelve patients each. Every ward opens on to long intercommunicating corridors. The male division has a superficial area of 14,973 square feet, a total cubic space of 254,540 cubic feet, and accommodation for 90 patients. The female division embraces an area of 9,588 square feet, a total cubic space of 164,542 cubic feet and can accommodate 70 inmates. Between the boundary walls and the hospital there is an intervening stretch of ground about 9 and 12 acres on the male and female wings respectively. Since 1920, the land on the male wing has undergone important developments which have a considerable bearing on the daily hospital life of the patients.

The staff of the Hospital is made up of the Resident Medical Officers of the Poor House, at present four in number, three Sisters of Charity, a Chaplain, a Ward Master, 19 male and 10 female nurses and attendants. The Resident Medical Officers, besides being in charge of the Leper Hospital, also perform all the professional and administrative duties of the Poor House and of the various smaller Institutions annexed to it. No one of the Resident Medical Officers is specially entrusted with the charge of the Leper Hospital.

A body which is closely associated with the Hospital is the Leprosy Board, composed of five eminent medical men. The Regulations in force enact that "the members of the Leprosy Board shall visit the Leper Hospital every two months to examine patients and attend to other professional matters". The Board is also entrusted with other functions, namely:

i) The examination of all reported or suspected cases, before admission into Hospital;

ii) the recommendation for discharge of patients in whom the disease is arrested, and for the continuance of anti-leprosy treatment as outdoor patients, when such treatment is advisable;

iii) the examination, every six months, of patients discharged from Hospital, of outdoor patients and of all contact cases.

On the opening of the Asylum, the Senior Resident Medical Officer of the Poor House and Leper Hospital formed part of the Leprosy Board, but later this arrangement had to be abandoned. The lepers showed much resentment against the members of the Board, whom they considered as the persons responsible for their internment. This resentment was mainly vented on the Senior Resident Medical Officer, the only member who came in continuous contact with the patients. Following the occurrence of repeated ugly incidents, directed towards the person of the Senior Resident Medical Officer, the Board was reconstituted and this Officer relieved of his duties in connection with it.

Concurrently with the opening of the Asylum, special regulations were issued. Under these rules, which in course of time have undergone extensive alterations and have been made less restrictive, lepers were absolutely separated from the outside world and were not allowed to communicate with relatives or friends, except on certain set days when they were permitted to see only their nearest relatives. The visitors were received in a special room divided by a grille, the patients standing on one side and the visitors on the other. Both patients and visitors strongly objected to this arrangement; as the complaint was just and the precaution practically unnecessary, the grille has since been removed, but an attendant is invariably present during visits. Patients who are dangerously ill may be visited in the ward at any time.

Under the regulations the same diet was allowed to the patients of the Leper Hospital as that prescribed to the inmates of the Poor House. Obviously, this diet was rather meagre, considering the state of health of most of the patients and the particular circumstances under which they were interned in the Institution. For these reasons the Medical Officers have always found it necessary to prescribe a more liberal diet. Additional food may also, within certain limits, be provided for the patients by their relatives or friends.

Personal articles of clothing may be used by the patients but all such clothing must be washed in the laundry of the Asylum. The taking out of hospital of any article whatever, used, worn or touched by the patients, is strictly prohibited.

The regulations also impose penalties in case of misbehaviour by the inmates, as follows:

i) prohibition of smoking;
ii) deprivation of the ration of wine or dessert; and
iii) confinement to their dormitory.

These punishments may be inflicted for:
i) violation of the regulations of the Institution;
ii) disregard of the orders of the Officials;
iii) creation of any disturbance;

iv) the use of obscene or profane language;
v) insolence or contempt against an official or another inmate;
vi) destruction of, or damage to, Government property or articles belonging to other inmates.

Any other offence which may fall under the Criminal Law of the Island is dealt with by the proper Court.

In March 1900, the male division was opened and the few advanced cases who were sheltered in a separate ward at the Poor House were transferred thereto. They numbered thirteen in all, which together with 68 other cases admitted during the year 1900, gave a total of 81 for the first year.

A notified case of leprosy is thoroughly examined by the Leprosy Board. If the person is certified to be suffering from the disease, under the Lepers Ordinance he is interned in the Leper Hospital. On the opening of the Asylum, a leper, certified as such, was there and then segregated, but as this procedure was somewhat too drastic and was strongly objected to, the provision was amended in the sense that a seven days' notice was henceforward to be given in each case and the leper interned at the expiration of that period.

As it may well be expected, the internment of lepers and the severe regime to which they were subjected, were the cause of very great unrest among the inmates, especially among those who were able-bodied and in the prime of life. They used every means in their power to have the law repealed; at least, partially to regain their freedom. Applications, petitions and protests were forwarded to the various civil and religious authorities. The Government, however, would not repeal or amend the law, and the regulations were not relaxed until some years after the opening of the Hospital. The refusal, on the part of the Government, to consider favourably their petitions aroused greater resentment among the lepers, and the first five or six years were marked by incessant complaints, frequent disturbances, escapes from Hospital and attacks on the personnel. This necessitated the retention of a detachment of police in the Hospital. On the removal of the police in 1903, the hospital attendants were given executive police powers. This circumstance was, of course, in itself sufficient further to irritate the inmates, and cases of insubordination occurred frequently. Offences against the ordinary law were dealt with by the Criminal Courts and several lepers were fined or imprisoned for inflicting personal injury, for breaking away from Hospital and for other crimes.

The Lepers Ordinance may seem to be harsh from the leper's point of view. The fact must not be lost sight of, however, that the law was enacted to safeguard the health of the community, the disease being contagious, especially through open sores and discharging lesions, which generally occur on exposed parts of the body. It is obvious that the danger of contagion is correspondingly greater if the occupation of a leper, having such lesions, entails his handling articles of food or clothing. It must further be understood that everything is done by the Government to accede to all reasonable requests on the part of inmates, and that no effort is spared to make their life as easy as possible. The families of lepers left unprovided for, are subsidized by the Government. The leper himself, who in most cases would be a burden to his family, is more comfortably housed and looked after than if he were living in his own home. Many of the patients are crippled, mutilated or disfigured. These considerations are quite sufficient to prove that the segregation of lepers in a well equipped hospital, besides being a desirable sanitary measure, is actually a humane method, in virtue of which the unhappy victim of leprosy is withdrawn from the battle of life, looked after by capable nurses and treated by experienced medical men.

It may be stated that, by the year 1907, the lepers had settled down to a normal life in the Hospital, and except for minor misdemeanours, which might and do happen in any Institution, no serious incidents ensued for a relevant period. In 1912 the female division was opened and 37 cases were admitted. Complaints of a new character had cropped up since 1910 among the male inmates, who alleged that the food and clothing supplied to them were deficient both in quality and in quantity. These complaints became intensified on the admission of the female patients, and minor acts of insubordination caused serious concern to the Government. In 1916, a Board composed of the Comptroller of Charitable Institutions, the Assistant Crown Advocate and the Superintendent of the Poor House and Leper Hospital, was appointed by Lord

Methuen, the Governor, "to enquire into the discipline of the Leper Asylum, and to recommend efficient measures for its proper maintenance, and to ascertain whether the inmates had any substantial grounds of complaint, and to suggest the means of removing any grievances that were well founded". The Board, in a lengthy and exhaustive report, gave an account of the indisciplinary acts of the inmates and brought to light very few real complaints; it was recorded that the manifold grievances brought before them by the lepers were unfounded and due solely to the exacting character of the patients themselves. Remedies were concurrently suggested to deal with the few actual grievances.

The contents of this report and certain opinions propounded at the time in the Island, regarding the low degree of communicability of leprosy, seem to have heightened interest in the disease, for two years after, (1918), a second Committee composed of the Chief Government Medical Officer, the Chief Justice, Colonel A. Garrod A.M.S., Dr. P.P. Debono and Dr. E. Meli, was appointed, also by Lord Methuen, "to study *de novo* the question of the seclusion of lepers enforced by the law". The Committee also dealt thoroughly with the subject, and reported at some length on the contagiousness of leprosy and on the advisability of drastic measures to check its spread. The Committee concurred in the opinion that the compulsory segregation ordinance then in force was the best and only method for the attainment of this end, but maintained that patients compulsorily segregated should have the right to all necessary comforts and to the best therapeutic treatment. Improvement of the study of leprosy was recommended, and several suggestions in order to ameliorate the lepers' lot were also made; most of these suggestions have since been adopted, while others are being gradually taken up.

An amended Lepers Ordinance was published in 1919, as a result of the report of the Committee, and, simultaneously, the regulations were revised, the main new provisions being the following:

    i) the grant of seven days grace after examination of a leper by the Leprosy Board, before internment;

    ii) facilities to patients to visit their sick relatives;

    iii) the discharge from Hospital of patients in whom the disease is arrested, and who are therefore no longer a danger to the public health. Patients discharged under this last provision are bound to inform the Authorities of their address and to present themselves every six months for examination by the Leprosy Board. They are, however, precluded from taking up certain particular trades and occupations.

Obviously, hospital life presents little or no difference from outdoor life to bed-ridden patients, but the internment of able-bodied men in an Institution throws them into a compulsory and deplorable state of idleness with consequent spare time on their hands to brood unduly over their misfortunes. The latter class of patients look upon the Hospital as a prison, into which they have been thrown through no fault of their own, just because they happen to be the unlucky victims of a horrible disease. Such morbid reflections, preying on the idle mind of the patients, naturally give rise to discontent, apathy, truculence,—all leading ultimately to disagreements, disputes, disturbances and other acts of insubordination. The Government has always done its utmost to make the life of lepers run as smoothly as possible; in order to lessen the acts of indiscipline and thus do away with punishments, a new scheme, suggested by the Committee of 1919, has been resorted to, with the object of diverting the mind of lepers from unhealthy introspection, breaking the monotony of their existence and their inactivity by work and exercise, and trying to encourage them to take an interest in hospital life.

The most important item for engaging the lepers' idle time is that of providing work. It is laid down in the revised regulations that "patients who are able to contribute some assistance to the service of the Institution or to perform agricultural, seamstress or other work, may be so employed in return to extra comforts or a small monthly gratuity". Thus, some of the patients assist the attendants in the cleaning of corridors, wards and hospital grounds; others work in the pantry, or in the Chapel, or as painters in the Hospital. In the case of female patients, besides assisting the attendants, sewing and darning are also done. The majority of the male patients, however, being skilled labourers, quarrymen and agriculturists, and there being a vast area of waste land around the Hospital, the plan of providing work for patients naturally extended itself to the reclaiming of that land. A sum of from £100 to £200 is voted annually by the Government in connection with this work, which was started in 1920. Since then, the waste land around the male division has been converted into fertile, beautifully laid out fields, which are cultivated by the patients. The crops are supplied to the Hospital and payment is made by the Government for these supplies, which are actually consumed by the inmates.

On the suggestion of the late Senior Assistant Superintendent (Dr. S. Marguerat), patients have also been allowed and encouraged to keep small poultry-farms away from the hospital premises, and this enterprise has assumed such proportions, that it has even been found possible for the Authorities to enter into regular contracts with patients for the supply of poultry and eggs to the Institution.

These schemes have turned out to be beneficial to the lepers in more ways than one. First and foremost, they serve the purpose for which they were originally intended, that is, to keep the patients busily engaged, and also to restore to the lepers some feeling of self-reliance. Secondly, the patients get an opportunity for physical exercise, which is one of the "five enemies of leprosy", (Muir). Thirdly, the patients derive therefrom financial profit.

It should be explained in this connection that the Government affords pecuniary relief to the families of lepers, in the shape of monthly subsidies, varying in amount in accordance with the earning capacity of the segregated member. The financial position of each family is also taken into consideration, but the relief is only granted if the interned member had formerly contributed towards the support of his family. Besides this subsidy, the actual travelling expenses incurred for visiting lepers, are refunded to near relatives when they happen to reside in certain outlying districts.

Under the 1893 Ordinance, and the provisions thereof, lepers were not permitted to leave the Hospital, except for one of the following reasons:
    i) to visit members of their family, physically incapable of travelling;
    ii) to leave the Island and establish their residence abroad;
    iii) to regain their freedom after being declared apparently cured by the Leprosy Board.

On special occasions, however, lepers have been granted special permission to leave the Hospital for a few hours; for instance, on the occasion of the purchase or the sale of land; for inspection of the sowing of crops, or the harvest; for drawing up contracts and for any other domestic, legal or financial transaction which may require the presence of the patient.

By 1901 the regulations had already been relaxed to such an extent that ablebodied inmates, two at a time, were being allowed to go out, under escort, for a walk in the country. In 1902 these walks developed into drives in a cart, exclusively kept for the purpose. In 1910 a cab was being used instead of a cart, and recently a char-a-bancs has been supplied, in which patients go for frequent drives to far off parts of the Island. This means of conveyance is highly appreciated by the patients, for they can enjoy the drive more, being a company of twelve every time; besides, they are enabled to get out of the Institution more often, and outings can be arranged in the country or by the sea-shore.

In their report of 1919, the members of the Committee fully explained the modern views regarding the low degree of communicability of leprosy. As a result of these conclusions, and following the recommendation of the Committee, lepers have been allowed a day out once every quarter, to visit their homes. They are accompanied by an attendant, who is given instructions as to the precautions to be taken by the patients, when in the bosom of their families. This concession, though first recommended in 1919, was only granted in 1929.

All sorts of amusements are arranged to while away the time for the inmates in the long evenings. A spacious room is used as a club-room, or as the lepers call it "il casin". A billiard table, a gramophone, musical instruments, dominoes and other indoor games are provided by the Government. For those able to read, papers and books in the vernacular, and English and Italian papers, both local and foreign, are obtained, besides novels, magazines and illustrated periodicals. The lepers are also permitted, within reason, to keep pets, such as dogs and canaries.

On certain special occasions during the year the inmates hold musical entertainments. Money is contributed by the patients for this object, and a few players and singers are engaged for the evening to entertain the patients with plays and songs, music and dancing. These entertainments have been a great success and cheer the lepers up considerably. The Government is contemplating the grant of a yearly subsidy for this purpose, and the purchase of a wireless set and a cinema apparatus.

***

The keen interest taken by Lord Methuen in the leprosy question in Malta was also shown by his successors in office (Lord Plumer and the late Sir Walter Congreve), and by the present Governor, Sir John Philip Du Cane, who has visited the Hospital on several occasions and has greatly interested himself in all matters affecting leprosy in the Islands. Ministers have also showed much concern, and have been unremitting in their efforts to make the life of the lepers easier and to keep the disease under control.

The many suggestions made by the Committee of 1919 for the improvement of the study and the treatment of leprosy, and especially the beneficial results obtained from the experimental studies of Dean, Mac Donald, Rogers and Muir in India with the Esters of Chaulmoogra and Hydnocarpus oils undoubtedly served as a great stimulus for the continuance of the struggle to eradicate leprosy from the Islands.

The outcome of the social interest taken in lepers has already been described. There now remains to be set down the therapeutic history.

On the opening of the Asylum, the crude Chaulmoogra oil constituted the only anti-leprosy treatment. It was administered orally, in drops or in capsules, but being very dense and nauseous, it was refused by the majority of the patients. Up to 1915, in the absence of a better treatment, the same unsatisfactory drug was still being used.

In 1915, Colonel Crofton, of the R.A.M.C., then in Malta, was given special facilities for the preparation of an auto-vaccine from the patients, who were given intravenous injections of the vaccine for fully two years. After this period the injections had to be stopped, for the patients refused to submit to further treatment on the ground that they derived little or no benefit from it.

From 1918 to 1923 six different preparations were tried. In the first three years of this period, use was made of "Collabiose Chaulmoogra", injections of which were given to 25 patients. The beneficial results obtained in India from "Sodium Morrhuate", aroused great hopes in the patients, and from 1920 to 1922, these injections were given to an exceptionally large number of 58 patients, who hailed this treatment with enthusiasm. The following preparations also had their share in the anti-leprosy treatment:—

i) A mixture of Esters of Acids of the Chaulmoogra series, known in the market as "Moogrol". (September/October 1922).

ii) An antimony compound, known as "Oscol Stibium". (November December 1922).

iii) "Cuprojodase" and "Cuprocian", both copper compounds. (January/February 1923).

In 1923 the Ethyl Esters of Chaulmoogra oil were introduced for the first time in the treatment of lepers in Malta. The E.T.O. ("Ethyl Esther Hydnocarpate, Thymol and Olive oil"), and the E.C.C.O. ("Ethyl Esther of Chaulmoogra, Creosote, Camphor and Olive oil") mixtures were used, the latter for a more protracted period than the former, and these were replaced in 1928 by the less irritating injections of "Alepol", (selected fractions of the Sodium salts of the lower melting point fatty acids of the Chaulmoogra series); this is being used today as a routine treatment.

"Karpotran", a copper preparation, and "Solganal", a gold compound, are given as an alternative remedy to those patients who refuse "Alepol" injections. "Avenyl", a mercury compound dissolved in Hydnocarpus oil, is used in complicated cases requiring mercury in addition to the ordinary treatment. With a view to having every patient treated, inmates who refuse injections, are given the fresh seed of "Hydnocarpus Wightiana", although little benefit is to be expected from such treatment.

The result of the treatment has not so far been very encouraging. This, however, cannot be attributed to the inefficiency of the drugs used, but rather to the reluctance and irregularity of the patients in submitting to the treatment. Patients, on admission, are generally very keen in following up the directions issued to them by the Medical Officer, but they always expect a cure in the space of a very few months, and as soon as this period elapses and no particular improvement is noticed by them, they become irregular in their attendance for treatment, and many of them ultimately abandon it altogether. This indifference is also provoked in them by some of the patients previously admitted, who had not benefited from the treatment.

It will be easily understood that the extraordinary refractoriness of the patients to medical advice constitutes a great handicap to the harassed Medical Officers. Besides being a disadvantage to the patients themselves, it is a serious obstacle to the obtaining of statistics and to the estimation of the relative efficiency of drugs.

In connection with leprosy treatment, an important provision has recently (1929) been added to the Lepers Ordinance of 1919, under which lepers presenting no contagious manifestations of the disease are subjected to treatment outside the Leper Hospital. This is a policy which has been adopted in many countries. It was recommended to the Government by the Leprosy Board, after the methods followed in various leprosy centres in Europe and other parts of the world had been studied. Mr. Frank Oldrieve, late Secretary of the British Empire Leprosy Relief Association, on a visit to the Leper Hospital during a short stay in Malta in 1926, strongly urged the Authorities to introduce this project. The new law was made operative from January 1930, and up to date five out-patients have received treatment. These are all new cases, who have never been interned. None of the lepers segregated at the Leper Hospital has been found to be in a fit state to receive outdoor treatment.

This law attempts to solve the problem of dealing with leprosy in its early stages, that is, of cases that are not contagious and therefore do not call for segregation, but which require treatment against the possibility of developing active signs of the affection. Moreover, it furnishes an incentive to those lepers, who, being in the initial stages of the disease would hide themselves away for fear of being segregated, to come forward spontaneously for treatment at a time when the disease may be arrested.

As has already been stated, one of the recommendations of the 1919 Committee was the improvement of the study and the early diagnosis of leprosy. With this end in view, the Government has provided a sum of money in order that a medical man may proceed to India and improve his knowledge of the disease at the School of Tropical Medicine of Calcutta.

The object of the Government in sending out this Medical Officer to the School of Tropical Medicine is that he shall have opportunities of studying the results of recent investigations in the disease, and therapeutic and laboratory technique in connection therewith, as also to familiarise himself with the way in which the main Leper Homes abroad are managed and administered.

Leper Hospital—Malta.,
April, 1930:
J. BUGEJA.

GENERAL GEOGRAPHICAL DATA OF THE MALTESE ISLANDS.

I. The Maltese Islands lie about 60 miles to the South of Sicily and about 180 miles to the North of Africa.

II. Malta: length, 17 miles; breath, 9 miles; area, 95 square miles.
Gozo: ,, 9 ,,   ,, $4\frac{1}{2}$,,   ,, 26 ,,   ,,
Comino: ,, $1\frac{1}{2}$,, ,, $1\frac{1}{4}$,,

III. Latitude: N. 35.

IV. Zone: Subtropical.

V. Climate: Temperate.

VI. Average Annual Rainfall, 21 inches.

VII. Population: Census 1921: 212,258.
Estimated present population: (31. 12. 1929): 232,832.

STATISTICS.

(From the opening of the men's division in 1900, and the women's section in 1912, to the end of December 1929).

A. Incidence of leprosy: Rate per mille in 1913, after female lepers were interned and segregation made general: 0.54
Rate per mille in 1929: ... 0.31

R 25

B. Number of lepers admitted into Hospital since the opening of the male section in 1900 and the female division in 1912:

Males: ... 264
Females ... 108

Total ... 372

C. Table showing movement of 372 cases admitted:

	Admitted	Discharged				Remaining in Hospital on 31st December, 1929
		cured	left Island	dead	Total	
Men	264	22	6	195	223	41
Women	108	24	—	53	77	31

D. Table showing age (on admission) of 372 lepers:

	Below 10	10–20	20–30	30–40	40–50	50–60	60–70	70–80	80 upw.
Men	1	31	73	54	49	28	18	8	2
Women ...	—	15	33	26	10	15	8	1	—
Total ...	1	46	106	80	59	43	26	9	2

Lowest age: 8   Highest age: 84.

E. Table showing occupation of 372 lepers:

Occupation	M	F	Total	Occupation	M	F	Total
Agricultural labourers ...	81	22	103	Beggars	4	2	6
Day labourers	47	—	47	Plasterers	4	—	4
Housewives	—	27	27	Carpenters and blacksmiths	4	—	4
Hawkers, petty vendors and shop-keepers ...	18	4	22	Soldiers and seamen ...	4	—	4
Stone masons	18	—	18	Students and clerks ...	4	—	4
Fishermen	16	—	16	Priests and nuns ..	2	1	3
Carters and cabmen ...	16	—	16	Other occupations ...	11	2	13
Coalheavers	15	—	15	No specified occupation...	14	16	30
Lacemakers, spinners and weavers	—	15	15				
Servants and housemaids	6	12	18				
Washerwomen and seamstresses	—	7	7		264	108	372

F. Table showing distribution of 372 lepers according to residence:—

Town or village	M	F	Total	Town or village	M	F	Total
MALTA.							
Curmi	30	8	38	Lia	—	1	1
Gargur	28	6	34	Crendi	1	—	1
Musta	21	13	34	Marsa	1	—	1
Zeitun	16	13	29	Micabiba	1	—	1
Naxaro	22	6	28	Calcara	1	—	1
Birchircara	15	9	24	Birzebbugia	—	1	1
Melleha	14	8	22	Imghieret (P. H.)	—	1	1
Zebbug	16	4	20				
Zabbar	15	4	19	GOZO.			
Hamrun	13	—	13				
Siggieui	8	2	10	Sannat	10	3	13
Tarxien	6	4	10	Nadur	6	2	8
Zurrico	6	3	9	Ghainsielem	6	2	8
Sliema	4	2	6	Xeuchia	3	1	4
St. Paul's Bay	4	2	6	San Laurenz	3	—	3
Misida	2	2	4	Kala	—	2	2
Rabato	1	3	4	Victoria	—	1	1
Valletta	2	1	3	Caccia	1	—	1
Asciak	2	1	3	Migiarro	1	—	1
Migiarro	1	2	3	Zebbug	1	—	1
Paula	1	1	2	Kercem	1	—	1
Floriana	1	—	1		264	108	372

G. Table showing a yearly return of lepers admitted into the Leper Hospital:

Year	Sex	Existing in previous year	Admitted	Died	Left the Island	Discharged cured	Remaining at the end of year
1900	M	—	81	12	—	—	69
1901	M	69	4	10	—	—	63
1902	M	63	3	4	—	—	62
1903	M	62	2	4	—	—	60
1904	M	60	6	4	—	—	62
1905	M	62	6	3	—	—	65
1906	M	65	1	3	—	—	63
1907	M	63	4	1	—	—	66
1908	M	66	4	3	—	2	65
1909	M	65	4	8	1	—	60
1910	M	60	3	5	—	—	58
1911	M	58	10	11	—	—	57
1912	M	57	4	7	—	—	54
1912	F	—	37	1	—	—	36
1913	M	54	20	11	—	—	63
1913	F	36	9	1	—	—	44
1914	M	63	13	13	—	1	62
1914	F	44	5	2	—	2	45
1915	M	62	8	7	—	—	63
1915	F	45	3	6	—	—	42
1916	M	63	7	4	—	—	66
1916	F	42	7	7	—	2	40
1917	M	66	14	13	—	—	67
1917	F	40	4	5	—	1	38
1918	M	67	8	5	1	—	69
1918	F	38	2	5	—	—	35
1919	M	69	8	11	—	5	61
1919	F	35	1	—	—	4	32
1920	M	61	6	10	—	6	51
1920	F	32	3	1	—	4	30
1921	M	51	2	7	—	—	46
1921	F	30	2	—	—	1	31
1922	M	46	5	4	1	1	45
1922	F	31	—	2	—	3	26
1923	M	45	7	6	1	—	45
1923	F	26	6	4	—	—	28
1924	M	45	6	10	—	1	40
1924	F	28	2	2	—	1	27
1925	M	40	3	5	—	6	32
1925	F	27	1	1	—	4	23
1926	M	32	8	3	—	—	37
1926	F	23	7	5	—	—	25
1927	M	37	2	2	—	—	37
1927	F	25	10	2	—	1	32
1928	M	37	8	3	1	—	41
1928	F	32	5	7	—	1	29
1929	M	41	7	6	1	—	41
1929	F	29	4	2	—	—	31

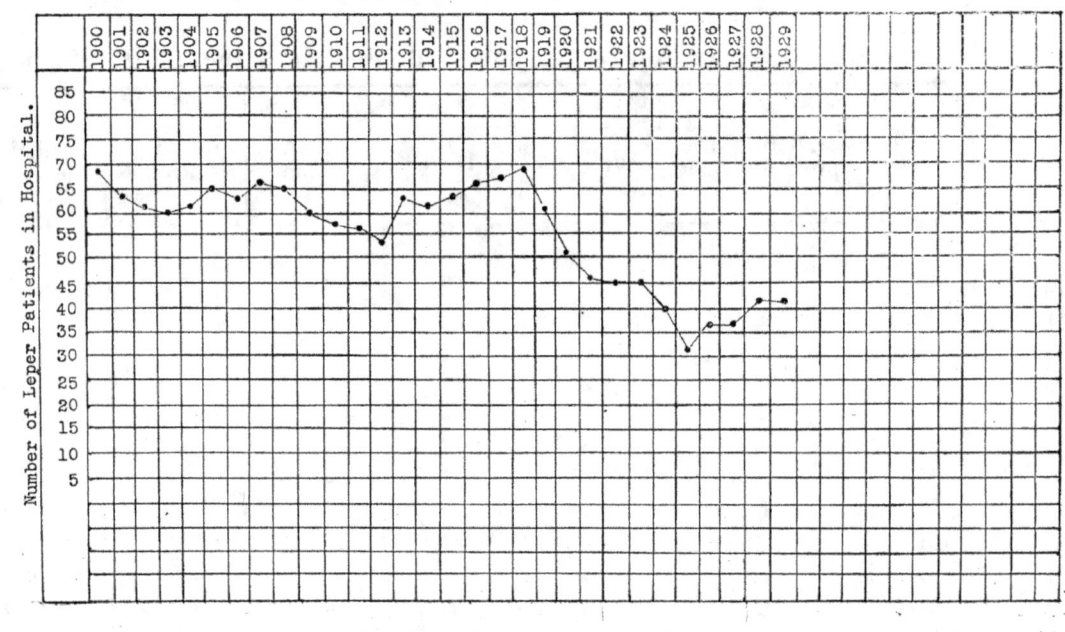

Graphic Representation of the Incidence of Leprosy for male cases admitted into the Leper Hospital from 1900 to 1929.

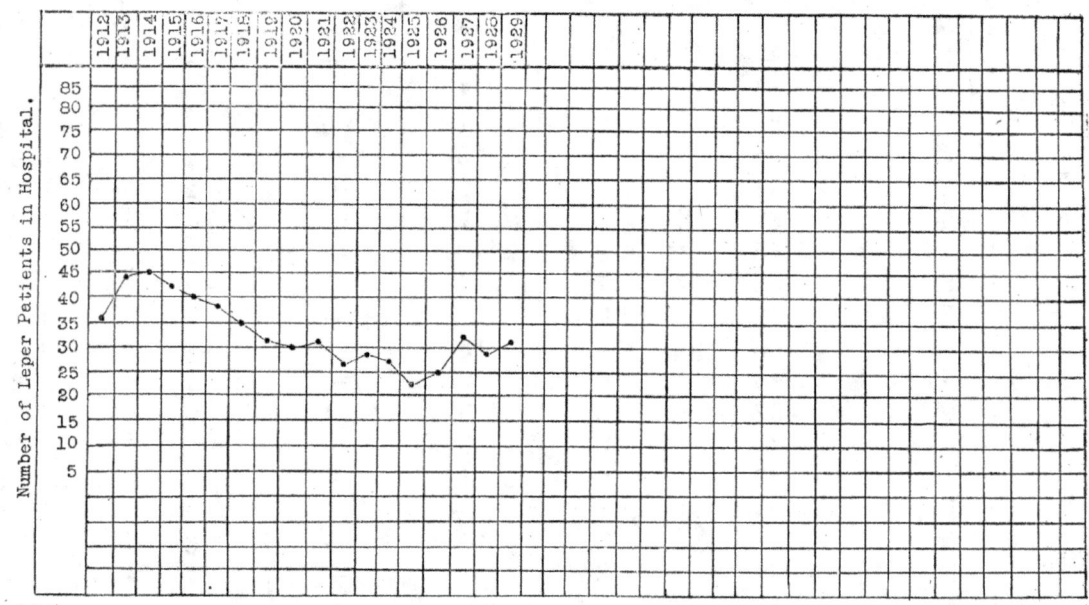

Graphic Representation of the Incidence of Leprosy for female cases admitted into the Leper Hospital from 1912 to 1928.

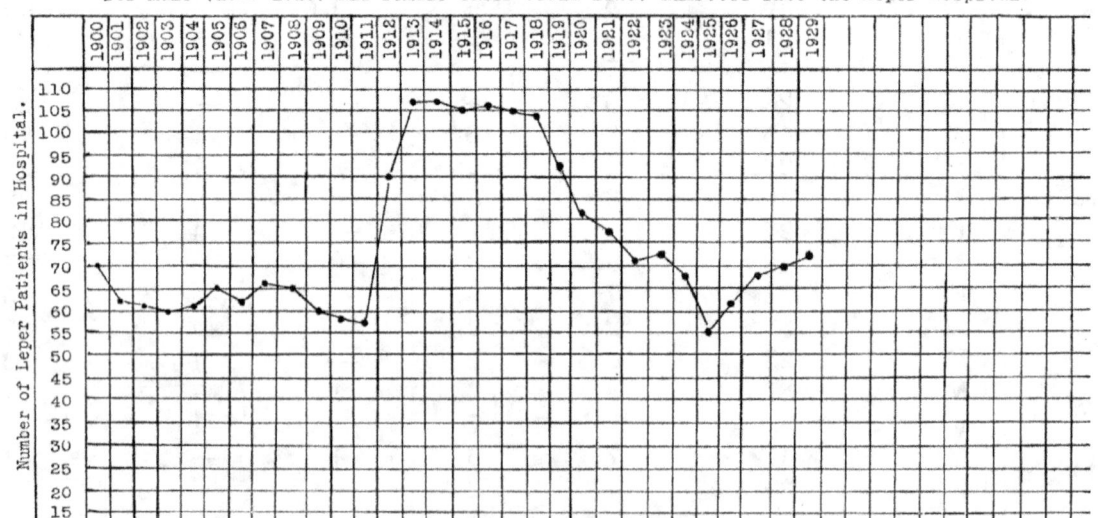

Graphic Representation of the Incidence of Leprosy for male (1900-1929) and female cases (1912-1929) admitted into the Leper Hospital.

LEPROSY IN MALTA

Professor Jos. Galea, M.B.E., M.D., D.P.H.,
Chief Government Medical Officer, Malta,
and
Dr. Edgar Bonnici, M.D.,
Medical Superintendent, St. Bartholomew Leprosy Hospital, Malta

Malta is the largest of a group of small islands situated in the middle of the Mediterranean. The aggregate area of the whole group is 121.8 square miles and the population is 314,369, with a density of 2,624 per square mile, one of the highest, if not the highest, in the world. The latitude is 35° N. and the longitude 14° E. The group of islands lies 60 miles south of Sicily and about 180 miles north of Africa and forms part of Europe. They enjoy temperate climate with an average annual rainfall of 21.5 inches.

Malta is the largest and most important of the islands. It is 17 miles long, 9 miles wide, with an area of 96 square miles. In its capital, Valetta, is the seat of the Government, and there is also the centre of the social, economic and industrial life of the Maltese archipelago.

Gozo, which is the second largest island, is 9 miles long, $4\frac{1}{2}$ miles wide, and covers an area of 26 square miles.

Comino, the smallest island of the group, is $1\frac{1}{2}$ miles long and $1\frac{1}{4}$ miles wide.

Almost half of the population live around the harbour, in urban areas where there are naval docks and some industries. The rest of the inhabitants are mostly engaged in agricultural pursuits.

The standard of living is of European pattern, the social services are advancing and the medical services have reached a high level. The general health is well maintained, no major infectious diseases have occurred for many years, and the only endemic disease is undulant fever.

Leprosy is one of the oldest diseases known on the face of the earth. The prejudice against the disease is such as to sever the victims from the sympathy and the society of other men. Both the Bible and the Koran contain references to the repugnance with which the disease was looked upon in olden times. The extraordinary **horror of leprosy** haunted ancient and modern men and engendered that sense of leprophobia which has been the bane of the wretched victims of the disease throughout the span of the ages.

Very little material is available on the history of leprosy in Malta; its origin is unknown, but it certainly existed in the island since remote times. It was suggested that the first cases were imported by the Phoenicians. Those sea-faring people, traders and colonizers, who came from the Near East, were the first historically recorded inhabitants of these islands. Malta was in the centre of their other possessions in the Mediterranean, owing to which position it became an emporium of a flourishing trade.

It is more probable, however, that the first cases of leprosy were introduced into these islands, in common with other countries on the Mediterranean littoral, during the Saracen domination between 870 and 1090 A.D., through the influx of leprosy-infected Arabs. In support of this contention is the fact that the only Maltese word meaning leprosy is " gdiem," pronounced " djem," the origin of which is from "judâm" or " djudhãm," the Arabic word for leprosy. The expansion of commerce and the migration of troops and mercenaries in the Middle Ages, an epoch in which war constituted one of the principal human activities, probably also played a part in the further diffusion of leprosy in these islands.

The early incidence of leprosy in Malta is obscure, but as far back as the year 1659 the disease must have been prevalent because on the 29th October on that year the Grand Master of the Order of Malta who ruled over the island, appointed a commission to provide for the care of sufferers from leprosy. On the 30th December, 1704, regulations were issued by the Chief Medical Officer of that time warning barbers against the dangers of accepting victims of leprosy as clients in their shops. From then onwards references to the disease were made from time to time in writings of medical men. By the second half of the nineteenth century the disease began to cause some anxiety among the population because in 1883 a committee composed of seven medical practitioners was appointed by the Governor " to investigate and study the incidence of the disease and to suggest means to check its spread."

Factors that no doubt had largely contributed to such an increase in the incidence of the disease were (i) the return of emigrants from countries in North Africa, where leprosy is known to be endemic, to which countries the Maltese had emigrated in large numbers during the economic depression that hit Malta between 1865 and 1872, and (ii) the stationing in Malta in 1878 of a strong contingent of Indian troops numbering over 6,000 men, in connection with the Russo-Turkish War. That this latter event had contributed largely to the increased incidence of leprosy in Malta can be seen from the earliest statistics which show that leprosy cases were most numerous in the villages lying near the place where the Indian troops had camped, the locality known as Imriehel.

In common with the policy then generally adopted in European countries, the Committee appointed in 1883 recommended that persons infected with leprosy should be compulsorily segregated. Other alternatives had been considered by the Committee before recommending segregation, but each had to be discarded. This accounts for the fact that it was only in 1893, that is after the lapse of 10 years from the appointment of such a Committee, that the first Leprosy Ordinance entitled ' An Ordinance for Checking the Spread of the Disease Commonly Known as Leprosy ' was enacted by the Local Government.

The Ordinance contained three main provisions, namely: (i) Compulsory notification of every case of leprosy immediately it became recognized by medical men and by certain other persons, namely, police officers, hotel keepers, etc.; (ii) Compulsory examination of each notified case by a Board of five experienced medical men (styled the Leprosy Board); (iii) Segregation of confirmed leprosy cases in a leprosarium so long as such cases were deemed to be a danger to the public health.

Segregation of confirmed cases in a leprosarium could not, however, be implemented immediately, as no special institution was as yet available for the housing of leprosy patients. A small number of patients in an advanced stage of the disease who had voluntarily applied for admission into an institution, were accommodated in a separate ward of the Asylum for the Aged and Incurables formerly known as the Poor House and now known as the St. Vincent de Paul Hospital.

Meanwhile the erection of a leprosarium was commenced in the locality known as Mgieret, an elevated site about 200 yards behind the St. Vincent de Paul Hospital. The male division was completed in 1900 and male patients were admitted and segregated therein. The female division, however, was not opened until 1912, when female patients were admitted and compulsory segregation was made general.

The Leprosy Hospital, known to-day as the St. Bartholomew Hospital, is a large and spacious building, having accommodation for the housing of 118 patients, i.e. 68 men and 50 women and about 40 staff. It is constructed on a plan of two lateral wings emerging at right angles from each side of a central block. The right wing is the male division, the left, the female division, while the central block, separating these two divisions, consists of the administration block, concert hall, dispensary kitchen and waiting rooms. With few exceptions, the patients are accommodated in the various wards in groups of from 4 to 10, according to the size of the ward.

Adjoining the hospital, stretching to the east and west of it and enclosed within high boundary walls, are plots of land, part of which is distributed into allotments for cultivation by the patients.

Following the repeal of compulsory segregation, the staff of the hospital at present consists of a resident medical superintendent who performs professional and administrative duties, three Sisters of Charity, a chaplain, a ward master, an assistant apothecary and clerk, 15 male and 9 female hospital attendants and 14 male and female domestic staff.

Concurrently with the opening of the leprosarium, special regulations were issued. Under these rules complete isolation from all contacts with society was enforced. Patients were permitted to see only their nearest relatives on certain days and in a special room. Only dangerously ill patients could be visited in the ward at any time. Such rules had undergone extensive alterations in the course of time.

As it may well be expected, this segregation of leprosy patients and the severe regime to which they were subjected, were the cause of discontent among the inmates and ugly incidents were of frequent occurrence. The hospital came to be regarded as a prison, with the result that patients suffering from leprosy were driven to secrecy and concealment.

Hence, it was only natural that, with few exceptions, only those leprosy patients in an advanced stage of the disease, who were hopeless and helpless, gave themselves up or were reported by their relatives, while those in whom the disease was in the initial stages, especially those who were able-bodied and in the prime of life, went into hiding in the countryside. Moreover, once leprosy patients were compulsorily segregated in hospital, it was difficult to obtain their co-operation with regard to treatment.

In the light of increasing knowledge, an amended Leprosy Ordinance was published in 1919. Compulsory segregation still remained the law, but patients in whom the disease had been arrested could, under this new amendment, be discharged from hospital. Patients so discharged were bound to present themselves every six months for examination by the Leprosy Board, and were precluded from taking certain trades and occupations.

In order to break the monotony of their stay in the institution and render life more bearable, provisions were made for each patient to be kept fully occupied in accordance with his inclination and capacity. Thus, patients who were able to assist in the domestic service of the hospital or to perform agricultural, tailoring, or other work, were so employed in return for a small monthly gratuity.

Govenment also afforded m netary relief to the families of leprosy patients in the form of monthly subsidies. Amusements were also organised to while away the time for the inmates in the long evenings.

A further amendment to the Leprosy Ordinance of 1919 was enacted in 1929 with a view to bringing the law into line with current trends then obtaining in Europe and in other parts of the world. Under the new bill, leprosy patients presenting no contagious manifestations of the disease were permitted to receive treatment as out-patients. By this new amendment it was hoped to induce the hitherto hidden early amenable cases of leprosy to come forward for treatment. The fear of compulsory segregation, however, still loomed in the minds of the majority of the sufferers from this disease, who were terrified by the thought that should the disease become infective at some later stage, they would lose their liberty.

The final blow to segregation was dealt in 1953 when the Leprosy Ordinance was again amended, abolishing the compulsory segregation of patients affected with leprosy and this method of prevention which in Malta had proved ineffective, came to an end.

The chief aim in abolishing segregation has been to attract early cases to come forward voluntarily for treatment. Previous experience has shrown that unless fear of compulsory segregation is dispelled from the minds of persons affected, the disease will remain difficult to control, as it will continue to be driven underground. As in tuberculosis, so in leprosy, the earlier in the course of the disease the treatment is instituted, the more hopeful will be the outlook for the patient; this is especially so nowadays when encouraging results have been obtained from sulphone therapy.

Under the new Leprosy Ordinance various sections of the principal law have been repealed, but cases of leprosy still have to be notified to the sanitary authorities by the medical practitioners, and certain precautionary measures have been retained. In exceptional cases segregation may still be enforced by the competent authorities under a different enactment, i.e. the Prevention of Disease Bill, when such a course is imperative, such as for example, in the case of a patient who persistently refuses regular treatment and does not avoid spreading the infection to other persons.

The new legislation was enacted with the object of attracting early cases to come forward for treatment, but at the same time it had the effect of diminishing the number of patients undergoing treatment in hospital. In fact many of the patients availed themselves of the liberty conceded by law and left the hospital. Other patients, however, were not in a position to ask for their discharge. Disfigurement, indifferent relatives, the absence of proper accommodation at home and above all straitened financial circumstances, will always keep a number of patients inside the hospital.

To alleviate the lot of these patients and to render their life in the hospital as pleasant as possible, immediate steps were taken to provide them with comfort and amenities. A new hospital coach has been provided and outings are being organized more frequently; facilities for regular home visits have been arranged; the tobacco allowance has been increased, and the remuneration for services rendered in the hospital has also been increased. Rediffusion sets have been provided both in the male and female divisions, and television sets are being installed. Cinema shows take place weekly and performances by local theatrical companies are given regularly. In addition generous cash allowances are granted monthly to families or dependents of leprosy patients undergoing treatment at the hospital.

Incidence and Anti-Leprosy Campaign

In 1913 when segregation was compulsory the incidence index for leprosy was 0.54 per thousand; the estimated civil population for that year being 216,617.

In 1930, the rate was 0.34 on an estimated civil population of 234,454.

In both instances the rate was based on the number of patients segregated in relation to the estimated population of the islands at that time. In the latter instance it took into account neither the number of patients who had been paroled under the amended Leprosy Ordinance of 1919, after having undergone treatment at the hospital, nor the number of leprosy cases on the official records of the Leprosy Board, who were suffering from leprosy in a non-infective stage and consequently not recommended for segregation, following the amended Leprosy Ordinance of 1929. Naturally no account could be taken of the number of patients in hiding.

The total number of registered cases of leprosy in Malta and Gozo as on December, 1956, was 144. This figure, on an estimated civil population of 314,369 gives a rate of 0.45 per thousand. In the absence of a detailed survey it is not possible to give an accurate figure of the number of cases of leprosy in these islands, but it is calculated that their number does not exceed 200, the rate per thousand being therefore approximately 0.64. All attempts to carry out a complete examination of contacts and other close relatives have in the past proved unsuccessful. The lepromatous rate is 66%

of all known cases, and the child rate in the 534 cases notified since 1920 is 3% (children under 15 years of age numbered 21).

As already stated, in order to induce patients and their contacts to come forward for treatment, generous grants have been instituted to the households of patients suffering from leprosy. Such generous grants will also help contact-families to raise their own resistance to infection by better feeding and housing.

Social assistance is given in some measure to all patients suffering from leprosy and also their dependents. However, those patients who are not undergoing treatment in the hospital must attend at regular intervals for examination and treatment at the Out-patients' Clinic to qualify for the assistance. Should they fail to attend regularly for treatment their allowance will be temporarily discontinued.

The health authorities spare no effort to encourage patients to come forward for treatment and to persuade contacts to report for periodical examination at the Clinic.

BCG vaccination is freely offered to all contacts of leprosy patients, particularly children.

Sanitary inspectors pay frequent visits to the homes of patients living outside the hospital and give instructions and advice as to the precautions to be taken in order to prevent or minimise the danger of spreading the infection. On the suggestion of the Medical and Health Department, the Housing Department has on occasions provided suitable accommodation for families in which leprosy has occurred.

Treatment

The use of chaulmoogra oil and its derivatives has long been abandoned in our hospital. Our experience is that patients did not derive much benefit from the use of these drugs, which frequently aggravated the condition of those patients suffering from the lepromatous type.

Although many different forms of treatment have been tried in our hospital, sulphone treatment in various forms has remained the standard treatment of leprosy. It is now nine years since sulphone treatment of leprosy was first introduced in our hospital, and since that time marked improvements have been noted, especially in the general health and clinical appearance of patients, the majority of whom are of the lepromatous type. Bacteriological improvement is, however, slow.

As we do not know whether the infection is ever eradicated from the patient, we continue to administer sulphone treatment

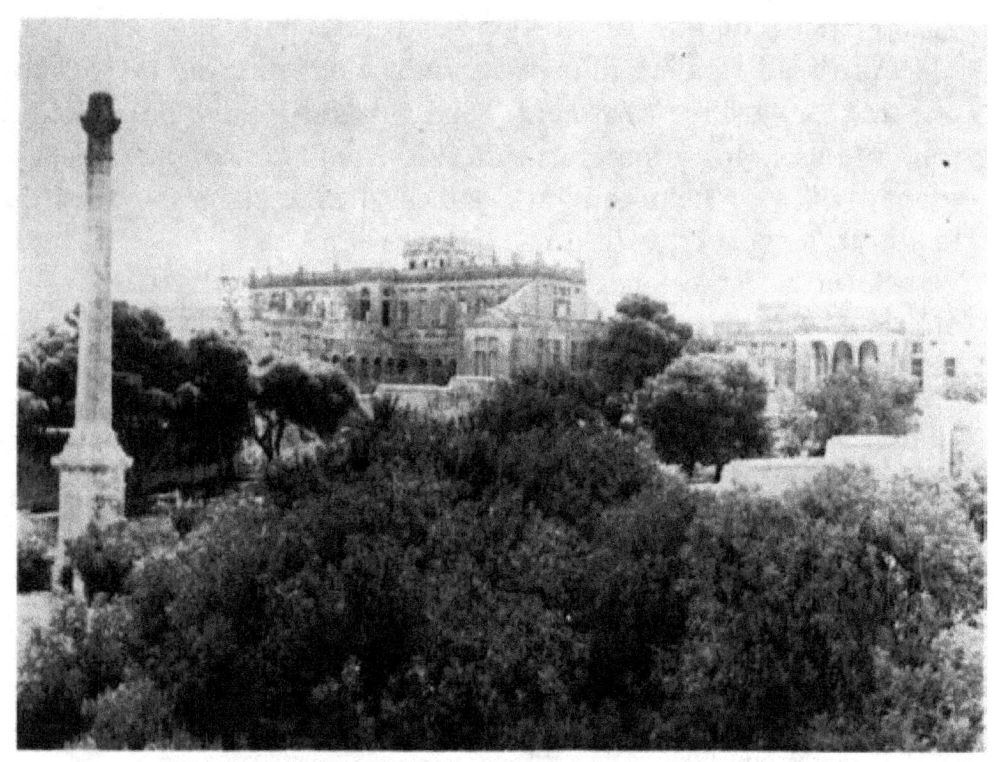
General view of St. Bartholomew's Leprosy Hospital

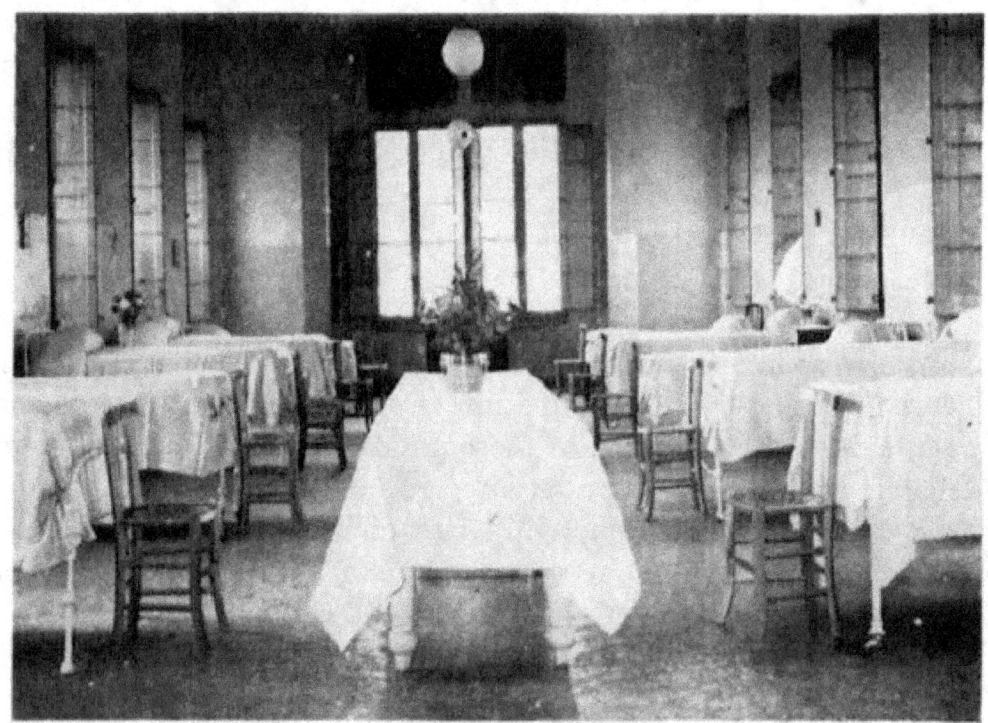
One of the larger wards

indefinitely, at reduced doses, even to those patients in whom the disease has been arrested.

On the whole, sulphones are well tolerated. Reactions from their use, such as erythema nodosum leproticum, mild mental derangement, etc., are occasionally met with. Such reactions subside after reduction of the dose or temporary withdrawal of the drug. Iron and yeast preparations are administered concurrently with sulphone treatment.

In common with all leprosy subjects of European descent, our patients in the past suffered extensively from eye and throat complications. Good results have been achieved from the local use of cortisone in leprotic eye complications. Leprotic blindness is now rare. Lepromatous laryngeal involvement, once so common among advanced lepromatous cases, is now extremely rare in patients undergoing treatment with sulphones. The death rate from leprosy has fallen also in recent times.

The government ophthalmologist visits the hospital at regular intervals to examine and treat the eye complications of the patients. The dermatologist pays frequent visits to the hospital in his capacity as senior leprologist. Leprosy patients who in the course of their disease develop some acute medical or surgical condition are admitted temporarily at St. Luke's General Hospital for the required treatment, and they are kept in separate wards. School medical officers are also instructed to look for the disease during their routine inspections of school children. No efforts are being spared in the teaching of young doctors how to diagnose the disease in its various phases.

Conclusion

The present trend in dealing with leprosy patients does not seem to favour compulsory segregation; this method is becoming obsolete; it has its utility as a check on the spread of disease, but it has also many drawbacks, social, ethical and administrative, and it certainly does not seem to agree with the modern outlook of thought and life. It has been ascertained that the ancient system of compulsory segregation may do more harm than good in causing the early cases to be hidden for fear of life-long imprisonment, until it is too late for effective treatment, and they have already infected members of the household. With the modern drugs and modern methods of treatment the course of the disease may be favourably modified, especially if patients seek medical advice early. Improved standards of living, better hygienic conditions, health education and adequate social services have also their beneficial effects.

BIBLIOGRAPHY

"International Congress for the Defence and Rehabilitation of the Leprous." Rome, April, 1956—Edizione Mediche e Scientifiche, Rome.

"Round the World of Leprosy," by R. V. Wardekar. Gandhi Memorial Leprosy Foundation, Wardha, N.P. India.

"Leprosy in the United States," by L. F. Badger. Trop. Dis. Bull., Vol. 53, No. 5, May, 1956. Abstract, p. 601.

"The Incidence and Epidemiology of Leprosy in Uganda," by J. A. K. Brown. Trop. Dis. Bull., Vol. 52, No. 9, Sept., 1955. Abstract, p. 903.

"Report of the Health Conditions of the Maltese Islands for the Year 19 Govt. Printing Office—Malta, 1954.

8. P. Cassar: Leprosy. In: *The Medical History of Malta*. Wellcome Historical Medical Library, London, 1965, p.210-217

9. C. Savona-Ventura: Hansen's Disease in Malta. *The Sunday Times (Malta)*, 29th January 1995, p.32-33

10. P. Cassar. A torch-bearer in the control of leprosy in Malta. *The Sunday Times (Malta)*, 26th February 1995: 59.

Medical historian Dr PAUL CASSAR recalls the figure of physician and poet Rużar Briffa, B.Sc., MD (1906-63), whose 32nd death anniversary fell last Wednesday

A torch-bearer in the control of leprosy in Malta

IN CONNECTION with the dedication of January 29 as World Leprosy Day it is appropriate to recall the figure of a Maltese torch-bearer in the treatment and control of leprosy in our islands – the physician and poet Dr Rużar Briffa.

Born in Valletta on January 16, 1906, Dr Briffa studied at the Lyceum and at the Medical School of our University. He obtained the Diploma of Pharmaceutical Chemist (Ph.C.) and the B.Sc. in 1928 and graduated in medicine in 1931. That same year he was awarded the Strachan Travelling Scholarship which enabled him to proceed to London where he followed an academic and practical course in the pathology and bacteriology of skin diseases at the Institute of Dermatology.

On his return to Malta in 1932 he was appointed houseman in the Skin Diseases Section of the Central Hospital, then the General Hospital of Malta, at Floriana.

During the plague epidemic of 1936-7 he served as Assistant Medical Officer at the Isolation Hospital on Manoel Island returning to the Central Hospital a year later as Assistant Medical Officer in charge of the Department of Skin and Sexually-Transmitted Diseases.

Following his appointment as Leprosy Control Officer in 1938, he went to India where he studied the manifestations and treatment of this illness at the Calcutta School of Tropical Medicine.

Leprosy has been recorded in Malta since 1630. Its possibility of being a communicable disease was officially recognised in 1679 when the isolation of affected persons was resorted to as a means of avoiding contact with healthy individuals. Emphasis on segregation was still prevalent by 1893 though provision for the institutional care of the patients came into being ten years previously.

This was the situation when Dr Briffa was appointed Leprosy Control Officer in 1938. He found that segregation had proved a stumbling block to the early treatment of the illness as, owing to the fear of segregation, leprosy sufferers, instead of seeking treatment, concealed the existence of their malady until this reached an advanced stage.

It was only in 1953 that Dr Briffa had the satisfaction of seeing the abolition of compulsory segregation. By then the number of leprosy sufferers in the Maltese Islands was estimated to be 151.

The writer recalls Dr Briffa's sensitivity of character in the face of the physical and psychological sufferings of his patients: his gentle and unharried bedside manners; and the ripple of a smile that lighted his usually sad countenance, when reassuring the most pitiful cases. He was no controversial person but a humble retiring man quite aware of the limitations of his specialty.

He faced the anxieties of his private life and the trials of his professional career with stoic equanimity. He dealt with the popular prejudices which militated against the specialties to which he had devoted himself – the treatment of sexually-transmitted diseases and leprosy – with unflinching determination and unswerving endeavour.

During World War II (1940-43) apart from his duties as Leprosy Control Officer Dr Briffa was appointed Medical Superintendent of the Blue Sisters Emergency Hospital for the reception of casualties from air bombardment in the Sliema and St Julian's areas.

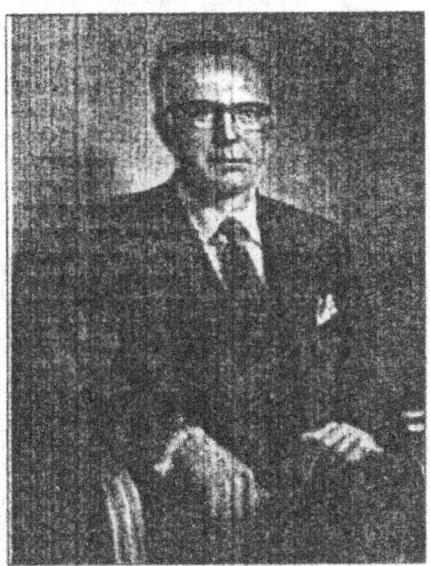

BRIFFA'S PORTRAIT at the Medical School, Guardamangia

Bibliography

1. *A Modern Crusade*, Palazzo Malta, Rome (1962), pp. 56, 58.
2. Briffa, R. "Pre-Cancerous Dermatoses" in *The Chest-Piece*, 1959, Vol. 1, pp. 6-8.
3. *Calendar for the Academic Year 1958-59*, The Royal University of Malta, Malta, 1958, p. 32.
4. Cassar, P. *The Control of Infectious Diseases in Malta*, Proceedings of the Seminar by the Union of Government Medical Doctors, Malta, January 25, 1992, pp. 7-14.
5. Cassar, P. *Medical History of Malta*, London, 1965, pp. 210-217.
6. Chetcuti, Ġ. *It-tabib Rużar Briffa*, *It-Torċa*, January 8, 1961.
7. Documents in the possession of Mrs L. Briffa.
8. Friggieri, O. *Rużar Briffa. Il-Poeżiji Miġbura*, Malta, 1983.
9. *The Times*, March 16, 1987, p. 13.

During World War II (1940-43) apart from his duties as Leprosy Control Officer Dr Briffa was appointed Medical Superintendent of the Blue Sisters Emergency Hospital for the reception of casualties from air bombardment in the Sliema and St Julian's areas.

In 1944 he was raised to the grade of Visiting Physician to St Bartholomew's Leper Hospital. With the return of normal peaceful conditions he went to Sicily to visit the *Reparto Dermo-Sifilopatico* in the General Hospital of Catania and the *Stazione Sanitaria Marittima* at Palermo, Catania and Syracuse (1949).

Following his appointment as Senior Consultant in Dermatology at the Central Hospital (1950) Dr Briffa attended a refresher course in skin diseases and leprology at the *Policlinico* of Rome. At this juncture (1950) he occupied the post of Lecturer in Dermatology and Leprology at the University – a post which he held until his death.

In 1959, in a review of a number of pre-cancerous skin conditions that had come under his observations, he pointed out the risks that could arise from exposure to X-rays, radium and the sun's rays. His wise warnings are still valid today.

His contributions to Maltese poetry – 32 years after his disappearance from the literary scene – continue to be read and appreciated by a young generation that did not know him personally. His contemporaries have commemorated his poetic gifts in various ways – a marble plaque (1971) at the University as co-founder of the *Għaqda tal-Malti (Università)* on the 40th anniversary of the foundation of this society; another plaque (1972) in the public garden of the Upper Barracca in Valletta; the issue of a postage stamp (1980) in the series of prominent Maltese personages; and in naming the new Head Office of the Mid-Med Bank at Qormi after him (1987) to honour, in the words of the bank chairman of the time, Rużar Briffa's standing "as a poet, his patriotism, his excellence as a doctor and the very humane way he went about his work"; and to inspire the staff of the bank to imitate these qualities in their dealings with the public.

By the time of his death on February 22, 1963, Dr Briffa's leading poetic status in Maltese literature had overshadowed his accomplishments in the field of medicine. It was only in 1973 that his merits as a protagonist in the fight against leprosy in Malta were recognised when the former St Bartholomew Hospital for Lepers was renamed Sptar Rużar Briffa and when a new wing at the nearby St Vincent de Paul Hospital

The greatest accolade that was ever bestowed upon him was the posthumous conferment of the decoration of the Sovereign Military Order of St John *Pro Merito Melitense* by the Prince and Grand Master and Council of that Order on August 2, 1988. The special significance of this honour stems from the fact that the care and welfare of lepers on an international scale is one of the main activities of the Order.

Quite recently his medical stature was acknowledged, this time by his academic colleagues, when his portrait, donated by his wife, Mrs Louisette Briffa, was added to the portrait gallery of the Medical School during a memorial ceremony held on May 21, 1994. That portrait is a vivid reminder to the present generation of physicians to look at him afresh in the context of the medical knowledge and the limited therapeutic tools of his time when results of therapy were not immediately visible and attained but had to be measured in years if not decades.

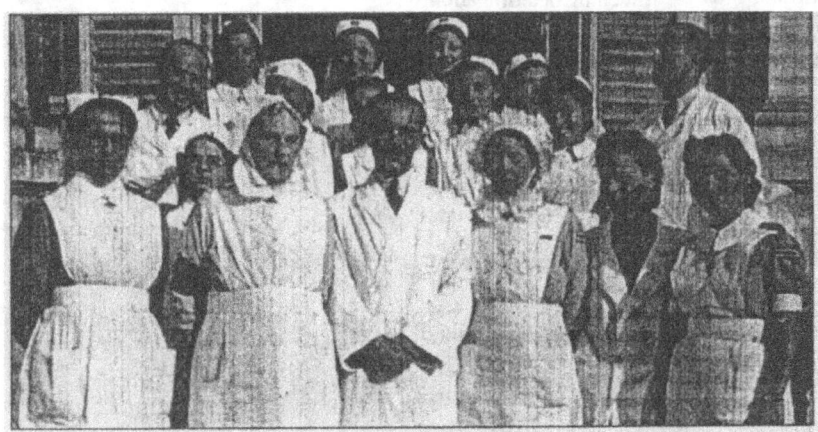

DR RUŻAR BRIFFA (centre) with his medical and nursing staffs at the Blue Sisters Emergency Hospital in 1940-43

11. B.M. Palmier: *Why did Hansen's Disease (Leprosy) in Malta persist until 2000 A.D.* Dissertation: Diploma in History of Medicine, Society of Apothecaries, U.K., 2003, +20p.

DISSERTATION

FOR THE DIPLOMA IN

THE HISTORY OF MEDICINE

OF THE SOCIETY OF APOTHECARIES

PRESENTED BY

DR. BERYL M. PALMIER

SEPTEMBER, 2003

I hereby certify that this dissertation entitled "Why did Hansen's Disease ("leprosy") persist in Malta until 2000 A.D. ?" is entirely my own work and I allocate joint copyright to the Society of Apothecaries.

September, 2003   *Beryl M. Palmier*
(Number of words: 4,702)

WHY DID HANSEN'S DISEASE ("LEPROSY") IN MALTA PERSIST UNTIL 2000 A.D.?

The first documented case of leprosy is recorded in the Archives of the Dominican Priory in Rabat. In 1629 the cost of a slave is recorded. The slave was bought in order that he should care for a friar, who was dying of leprosy[1].

In view of the lack of documentation and the uncertainties of diagnosis prior to the 19th century, I will confine my dissertation to the period subsequent to the time of the arrival of the British in 1800. . Initially I will enumerate the relevant factors and then deal with them in detail.

RELEVANT FACTORS

1. Position of Malta in the Mediterranean
2. Size and density of population
3. Original source of infection, and definite likelihood of sources of re-infection from outside Malta
4. Persistence of leprosy, despite plague and cholera epidemics.
5. Poverty during the 19th Century
6. Insanitary conditions in 19th and early 20th centuries.
7. Marked leprophobia and taboo.
8. The incubation period.
9. The type of leprosy.
10. Segregation and the aftermath.
11. No effective treatment until 1972
12. Policy with regard to children.
13. Genetic factors

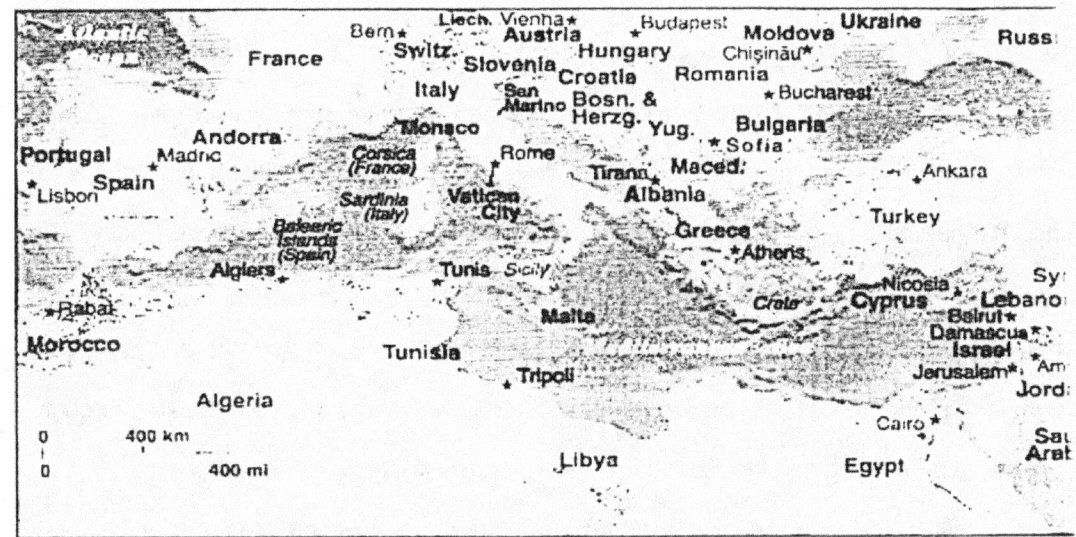
STRATEGIC POSITION OF MALTA IN MEDITERRANEAN

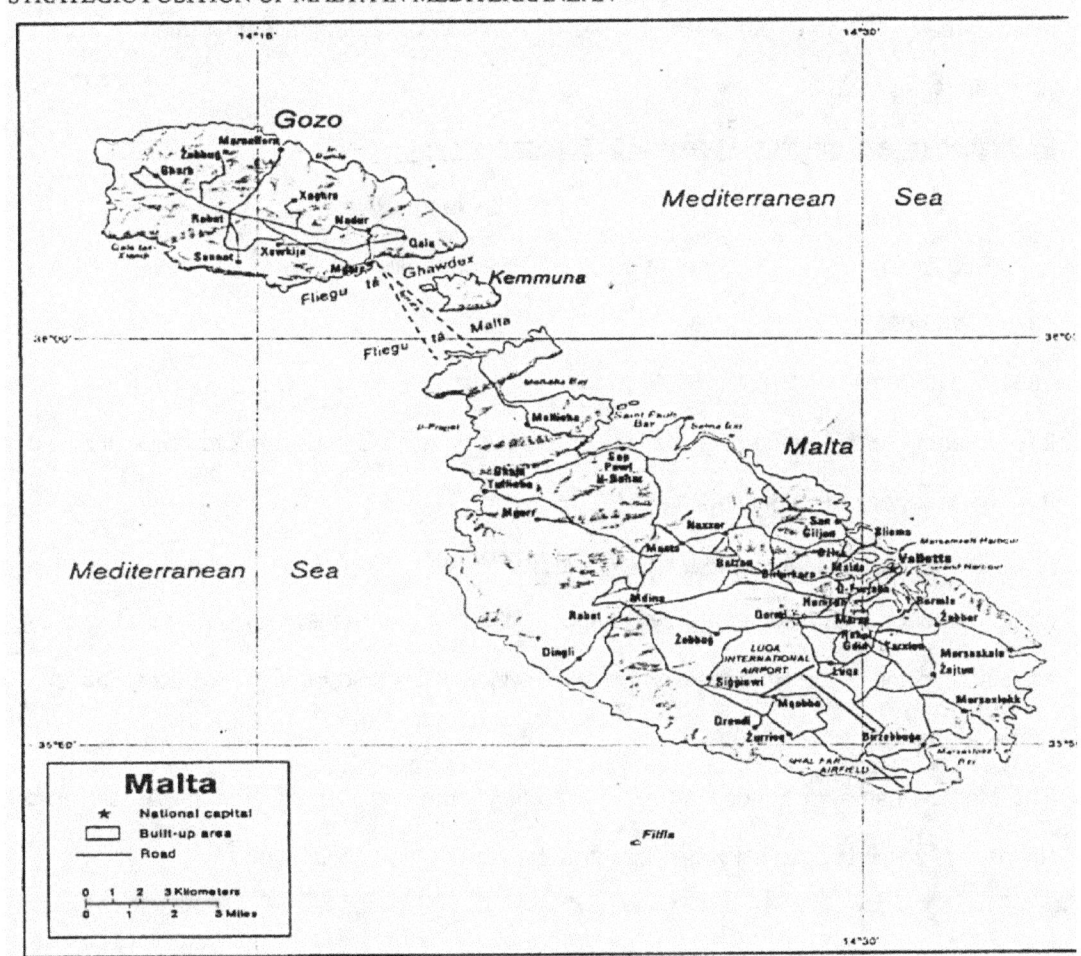
THE ISLANDS OF MALTA, GOZO AND COMINO (KEMMUNA)

POSITION OF MALTA (See Maps on Page 2)

35.50 North 14.35 East. 180 miles from Africa and 60 miles from Sicily.. It is in a very strategic position – approximately midway between Alexandria and Gibraltar with one of the best harbours in the Mediterranean. It has been on the trade routes since Phoenician and Roman Times and was a centre for the slave trade..

The opening of the Suez Canal in 1869 led to more traffic through the Mediterranean and a faster link for the passage of troops to India. The greater the numbers passing through especially from Africa and the East, the greater the risk of infections of all types.

Size of Maltese Islands :Approximate maximum lengths and widths. Malta: 17 miles by 8 miles (Area of 122 sq miles) Gozo: 9 miles by 4 ½ miles. (26 sq, miles) Comino: 1 ½ by 1 ¼ miles (1 sq mile).

Population (one of the highest density in Europe)[2]

Year	Malta Population	Density per sq. mile	England & Wales Density per sq. mile
1871	149,000	1,006	389
1951	313,000	2,115	750

It is generally accepted that high density of population assists the spread of epidemics and the maintenance of foci of infection.

ORIGINAL SOURCE OF INFECTION WITH LEPROSY

Malta has been occupied serially by 8 nations. It is thought that leprosy was introduced by the Phoenicians or the Romans who travelled widely. It is said to have existed at the time of the Arabs (870 AD – 1090 AD)

The Maltese name for leprosy is "djem" or "gdiem", the origin of which is the Arabic word "djudsam", which suggests it was present at the time of their occupation.[3]

3

The Knights of St. John record that they had segregation of leprosy cases in Rhodes where leprosy was quite prevalent. It is likely that they introduced it into Malta in 1530. They brought with them from Rhodes the right foot of St. Lazarus (no doubt, as a preventative and curative!!).[4]

Definite Likelihood of Sources of Re-infection from outside Malta

1872 Many Maltese settlers returned from North Africa where leprosy was endemic They had emigrated during the economic depression in 1865-72.[5]

1878 6,000 Indian troops were stationed at Imriehel.(They were reviewed by the Duke of Cambridge, whose verdict was "fine body of men with charming horses"!!) Following this, cases of leprosy started to increase in frequency in the villages of Qormi, Mosta, Zebbug and Naxxar[6](see Map on Page 2) close to this area.

1917 Committee reporting to H.E. Governor stated that the maximum notifications of leprosy for the previous year were still from these villages; % person with leprosy to total population in those villages was 39.75% whereas in the Inner Harbour area it was only 1.60% .[7]

1882 Following the massacre in Egypt by the rebels led by Ahmed Arabi, thousands fled to Malta including 6,632 destitute Europeans.[8]

1911 1,300 refugees arrived from Tripoli, when it was occupied by the Turks during the Italo-Turkish War. Many of them were Maltese.[9]

1915-1917 Malta was the "Nurse of the Mediterranean" The sick and wounded were accommodated in 25,000 beds in 27 hospitals (many buildings commandeered) A convalescent camp was set up for 4.000 and a further 500 convalescents were sent to Gozo.[10]

1916 1,670 prisoners of war from Bulgaria, Turkey, Austria and Greece were also accommodated.

Leprosy persisted despite epidemics

One of the common theories concerning the disappearance of leprosy in England after the 14th. Century was that the occurrence of the Black Death had killed all patients already weakened by leprosy.

Epidemics of plague have occurred with regularity in Malta. For example: in 1348 (when the mortality rate was 25%) also in 1427/8, and 1453. In the 16th and 17th Centuries there were 8 epidemics and 4 in 1813/4. Further outbreaks occurred in 1917, 1936/7 and finally 5 cases in 1945/6[11]. The plague in Malta was localised, mainly in the cities so foci of leprosy could persist.

Cholera

No "proven" case of cholera occurred in Malta until the world-wide pandemic in 1837.. There were 8 epidemics of cholera in the 19th. Century. The epidemic of 1911 had a mortality rate of 73%[12].

Leprosy continued in Malta despite these epidemics. It is likely that families were hiding leprosy cases so that they were effectively isolated from other infections.

1800 - Arrival of the British.

1867 The Colonial Secretary requested the Royal College of Physicians (London) to launch "An Inquiry into Leprosy in the Colonies". Malta was not mentioned in its report[13]!!

1867 The Maltese Government appointed a Medical Commission to inquire into the incidence of leprosy in Malta. Their verdict was that there was none! The explanation is uncertain.

POVERTY and POOR STANDARD of HEALTH

In many countries (e.g. Norway) this is correlated with the incidence of leprosy.

In 1868 a committee was set up to "Report on Distress".[14]

Unemployment was concluded to be the main cause.

5

War was always Malta's boom time, and in peace time there was recession.

184 workers had been "laid off" by the Military, Naval and Government Services.

419 mainly agricultural workers were out of work. Cultivation had been suspended due to the cholera and 3 years drought. The price of water had risen due to the cholera. (at this time it was necessary to import water from Sicily)

Maltese Lace had become fashionable after the Great Exhibition of 1851 and reached its peak in 1864. Following this, there was a decline which affected many who had been involved in this industry.

Despite the opening of the Suez Canal, in 1869, other circumstances adversely affected trade. Conditions deteriorated as was shown by:

1873 - Death rate of 23.39 per 1,000 population of Malta and Gozo

1874- Death rate of 49.24 per 1,000 population of Malta only (compared with the death rate in England of 22 per 1,000 population in urban areas and 19 per 1000 population in rural areas)

The Governor appointed a Commission whose task was to "Inquire into and report upon the causes of the recent increase in mortality in Malta". [15]

The committee's main findings were as follows.

Many men were working abroad. Prices had risen but wages remained the same. Infants were often left unattended while women worked in the fields. Mothers were ill fed, their milk failed and they attempted to give small babies solids.

Crops were deficient due to the high price of seed, increase in the price of land and climatic irregularities.

Unemployment was due partly to the fact that steam ships required fewer sailors, and the demand for sails and sailcloth had fallen dramatically with the advent of steam.

Sanitation, Sewerage, drainage and Water Supply.

Water supply in rural areas was from tanks filled from surface overflow from the open highways. The water was impregnated with impurities including "animal infusoria".

In the cities of Valletta and Floriana, the cisterns in the rock under the houses and palaces were filled by conduits from the 1616 Wignacourt aqueduct and Senglea, Cospicua and Vittoriosa were served by an aqueduct from Fawwara. These cisterns, which caused the walls of the buildings to be constantly damp, were often contaminated by infiltrating percolations from cesspits on higher levels.

Sewers and Inhygienic Conditions

In the cities, the connecting channels to the street sewers were often blocked. These were open to the atmosphere by vents which caused foul pollution of the air.

The police prosecuted those who threw raw sewage into the street, but the habit persisted in the poorer quarters[16].

The sewage was discharged, untreated, into the creeks that surrounded the cities.

Almost all the villages had neither sewers nor drains, Cesspits were emptied periodically, and the contents were stored in a small room in the corner of the yard. When dry, this was mixed with straw and used as manure. The pigs and fowl shared this yard, and all the family slept in one room, where there were no windows, only small vents in the wall facing the courtyard..

Similar living quarters existed for the poor in the cities; one room for all purposes!

In view of the high percentage of positive nasal smears in lepromatous leprosy, these conditions would lend themselves to making leprosy a "family disease".[17] There is also increased likelihood of physical contact, the other form of transmission.

7

Remedies suggested by the 1874 Commission were as follows.

1. Establishment of crèches in the villages
2. Improvement in sanitation
3. Separate accommodation for animals
4. Emigration to ease overcrowding and unemployment

Sanitary Reform

As a result of the 1874 Commissioners' report, large expenditure on sewage, drainage and the establishment of Public Health departments was undertaken.[18]

Dr. L. Leiker in his 1986 paper[19] felt that the decline in leprosy was closely linked with urbanisation and the improved socio-economic conditions.

TABOO AND LEPROPHOBIA

The Bible and the Koran contain references to the extraordinary horror with which the ancients regarded leprosy, and, no doubt have a bearing on the marked leprophobia which existed in Malta. Leprosy's unpleasant appearance and its incurability make this phobia understandable.

In Malta, any family with leprosy would be ostracised. Their livelihood could be threatened and their daughters' marriage prospects would be blighted. It was commonly thought to be hereditary. Affected relatives were hidden and there was great secrecy.

.Children were often unaware that their parents had had leprosy, even after the parents' death.(verbal communication Dr Depasquale). Brothers might be unaware that they each had leprosy. People with elevated social positions would resort to subterfuge to avoid their leprosy being notified, and some would go to England for treatment.[20]

Taboo led to delay in treatment. As cases were hidden, the incidence statistics were misleading. The following up of contacts and treatment of sub-clinical cases was impossible.

8

INCUBATION PERIOD

It is well known that this can be as long as 15 years. Dr Depasquale related an extreme case of a family, where the mother died of unknown causes, and the father died of leprosy. When the elder son developed leprosy, his younger sister was adopted by a neighbouring family. She completely lost sight of her blood relations. 35 years later she developed signs of leprosy. No alternative source was ever found.

The long incubation period makes this disease difficult to control, and sporadic cases will no doubt occur from time to time. Meanwhile it is well under control, and has been eradicated to all intents and purposes.

TYPE OF LEPROSY

77% of Leprosy in Malta was lepromatous. This has great bearing on the persistence of the disease as it is the most infectious.[21][22]

SEGREGATION

1886 Report of the Medical Committee appointed by the Government concluded that leprosy was confined to certain rural areas. Isolation was recommended

The occupations of persons with leprosy (bakers, pasta makers, cooks, shopkeepers and milkmen) resulted in their having contact with the population. Leprosy was especially prevalent among shop-keepers and hawkers.

1890 The Comptroller of Charitable Institutions advised the Government to legislate to check the spread of leprosy.

1893 Ordinance No. VII [23] dealt with compulsory notification and isolation. It was an offence to harbour persons with leprosy with intent to conceal or prevent their removal to the Asylum. The only way to avoid detention was to go abroad!!

Medical examination by Warrant, took place before detention in the Asylum

1897 1st. International Leprosy Congress and the 5th. In 1948 recommended isolation for infectious cases in leprosaria.

9

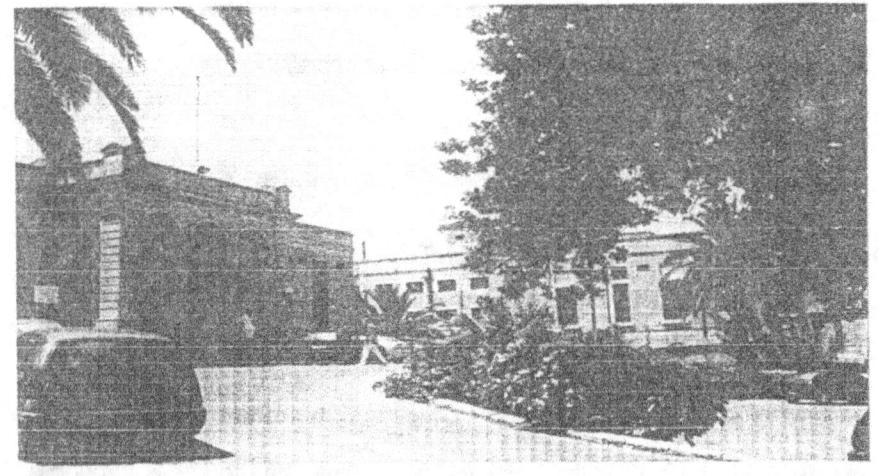
Leprosarium (subsequently named St. Bartholomew's Hospital) Main Entrance

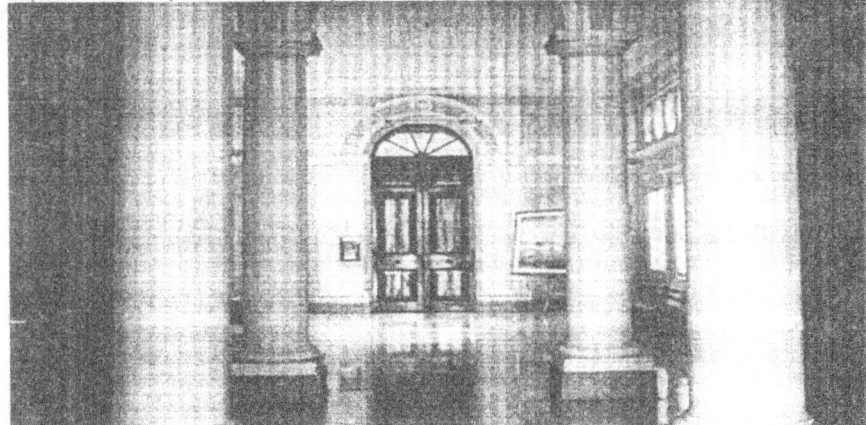
Leprosarium (St. Bartholomew's) - Entrance Hall with chapel entrance

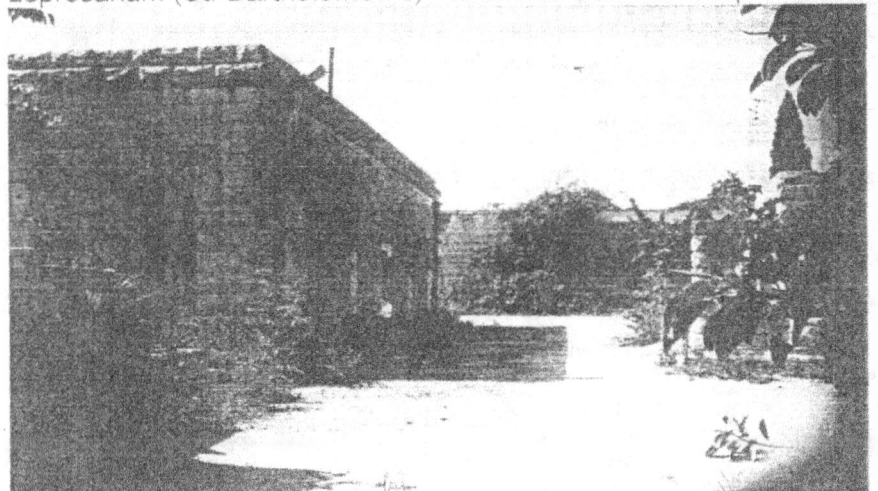
Community Building at Ferha – occupied when St. Bartholomew's closed and used 2001

Discussion as to site for the Leprosarium took into consideration that the patients might be there for the rest of their lives, so it must be reasonably comfortable.

The Male Division was occupied in 1900 and the Female Division in 1912[24]

The building consisted of a central block with the main entrance, the administration offices, chapel, the residences of the 3 Sisters of Charity (the Nursing staff) and the chaplain; the dispensary, stores, kitchen and laundry. On either side were the 2 wings, one for the men and one for the women. Wards contained 4 – 12 beds each, accommodating a total of 90 male and 70 female patients. There was a boundary wall enclosing 9 -12 acres. (see photos). Initially any visiting relatives had to speak through a grille similar to one in a cloistered convent

STAFF

Chief Medical Officer's jurisdiction initially extended to the Poor House. The animosity toward the Leprosy Board was so great that the CMO. had to cease being a member of the Leprosy Board. Later a separate Medical Superintendent of the Leprosarium was appointed, who had to have special training.

Four Resident Medical Officers also worked in the poor house.

Assistant Apothecary, Three Sisters of Charity , Chaplain, Ward Master, 29 Nurses (Male & Female) & Attendants

LAUNDRY No clothing was allowed to pass out of the hospital, it was all washed on site.

PUNISHMENTS e.g. no smoking, no ration of wine or dessert and confinement to dormitory were imposed for breach of rules, profane language and damage to Government property.

RIOTS

On two occasions in 1900 there was violence when the male patients forced their way out!! Furniture and windows were broken. In 1902 the Medical Superintendent had to leave as

11

the police could not keep order. After this disturbance two police constables were permanently on duty, and attendants were granted some policing powers.

MEASURES TO EASE THE TENSION

Financial aid was given to the relatives.

Occupational therapy was started: household or garden duties with small salaries.

From 1901 inmates were allowed to go out in twos for country walks. From 1902 they were allowed to be driven in a cart. From 1910 they were allowed cab drives.[25]

In 1916 the situation must still have been unsatisfactory because the Governor appointed a Committee in that year to study the question of seclusion and investigate complaints.[26] Its report in 1917 resulted in the 1919 Law. being passed to try and ease the situation. The committee recommended that a visiting physician should be appointed to study the disease abroad and a Government Travelling Fellowship instituted for a Medical Officer to attend the Indian School of Tropical Medicine in Calcutta. Other recommendations were for a course of instruction for local medical practitioners and the setting up of a research laboratory.

Incidence of leprosy based on patients segregated (per 1,000 of population)[27]

1913 it was 0.54 i.e. 117 cases out of a Maltese population of 216,617

1930 it was 0.34 i.e. 80 cases out of a Maltese population of 234,454

31% of the cases occurred in agricultural workers and the majority of patients were working class. The fact that the majority of patients were poor, made isolation in their own homes impractical.

1919 Law passed modifying 1893 Ordinance VII. This decreed the setting up of the Leprosy Board consisting of 5 eminent medical men who would pay visits every 2 months to the leper hospital and carry out:

(1) Examination of new admissions

(2) Recommendation for discharge of non-infectious cases on condition that they continued with anti-leprosy treatment as outpatients and attended regularly. They were precluded from certain trades.

(3) Six monthly out-patient examinations of: patients following their discharge and of their contacts.

<u>1919 Committee Recommendations - Relaxation of Regulations (to make the patients' life more tolerable)</u>

1. Confirmation of delay of 7 days after notification before segregation.

2. Facilities for patients to visit sick relatives

3. Work & exercise:

    Patients were encouraged to help run the hospital with cleaning, as seamstresses and in the kitchen.

    Men were allowed to reclaim land in order to grow crops and to farm poultry – this was so successful that poultry was supplied to the hospital under contract!

4. Patients were allowed leave for limited periods for special reasons e.g. to witness legal documents, buy land, inspect crops, or to go abroad !!

5. Entertainments organised: Clubrooms, Billiards, Cinema, Music, Library, Newspapers. Pets, e.g. dogs and canaries, were allowed. A special area was reserved for sea bathing.

1929 Act XV   Examination of contacts. Further relaxation of the rules.

1930 New cases not necessarily admitted to the hospital but treated as out patients if not infectious. Outpatients were allowed to travel by bus.

1937 <u>Leprosy Control Officer was appointed</u> to take control of all preventative measures e.g. follow-up of contacts, family welfare, education , etc

<u>A leprosarium was opened on the Island of Gozo</u> in Fort Chambray and called the Sacred Heart Hospital.

13

1938 The Malta leprosarium was renamed St. Bartholomew's Hospital to remove the stigma and given its separate organisation. (Previously it had been part of the Poor House Administration)

1938 Sir Walter Johnson following his medical inspection in Malta, (in consequence of 14 deaths from leprosy in 1936) requested the Medical Secretary of the British Empire Leprosy Relief Association, Dr Ernest Muir, to visit Malta and advise.[28] Dr Muir had a conference with the Lieutenant Governor. Firstly he stressed that leprosy should be regarded as a disease like any other and emphasis must be placed on the fact that it is less infectious than TB. Isolation must be achieved by cheerful co-operation. He reiterated many of the recommendations of the 1919 Committee that did not seem to have been put into action. He advised a leprosy survey, appointment of two leprosy experts, one for the hospital and one for village control with special treatment in endemic areas. He recommended the appointment of a lay worker to befriend the patients and organise their leisure activities

The Chief Medical Officer had not previously been a member of the Leprosy Board. Dr Muir felt that the CMO should be in control of the management of leprosy, and could be assisted by a small board of experts.

Staff for Educative Programme:

These must be experienced and keen. Dr Muir suggested that doctors with special leprosy experience in India should conduct a course specially aimed at doctors from areas with leprosy foci. Under this doctor's supervision local treatment of leprosy could be carried out by local doctors.

1953 Ordinance XI repealed Ordinance VII of 1893.

Segregation had been found to be counter-productive so countermanded. Only infectious cases to be persuaded to remain as In-Patients. Compulsory segregation now to be imposed only in certain circumstances.

14

St. Bartholomew's Hospital report for 1964:[29]

	Males	Females	Total
Out patient attendance	519	194	713
In patient attendance	23	19	42
Admissions *	3	0	3

* All readmission cases, though still active they had been discharged at their own request in previous years.

Discharges -			
at own request	2		2
died of nephritis		1	1

Ophthalmic referrals –
chronic dacrocystitis, cataracts and corneal ulcers – all successfully treated.
Type of Leprosy – vast majority were lepromatous.

1974 St. Bartholomew's closed and became an extension to the Old Peoples Home.

Tal Ferha Estate (see photo on Page 10) was opened for the remaining 22 cases in an ex-Army Battery. Each resident had a self-contained flat. They were allotted land in which to grow crops which generated income and were allowed to bequeath this land to a fellow inmate. They kept animals and cooked for themselves. There was a nurse on duty and doctors on call. Six-monthly checks were continued by the Leprologists.

1987 Six residents with an average age of 67 remained. Some had been admitted at the age of 18!!!

1999 – 2000. Three of the four remaining inmates died.

2001 The one remaining inmate was transferred to St. Vincent de Paul and the building was closed.

Effect of Treatment

The motivation of the patients to report their illness is, to a great extent, determined by the availability of effective treatment but initially there was none.

15

Chaulmoogra Oil 1900 – 1915[30]: Initially given by mouth and extremely nauseous. Many patients refused to take it. (So many escaped that escaping was made a criminal offence). Next it was administered intramuscularly. This was painful and not very effective. It had to be continued long term and patients lost heart, when they failed to see much improvement. In 1923 ethinyl esters of chaulmoogra oil were developed which made the injection less painful.

BCG was frequently offered to all contacts especially children but it was not given systematically in Malta.[31]

1955 Sulphones were first given in Malta .These were effective and inexpensive. Dapsone particularly had few side effects. .Sulphones were bacteriostatic only and very slow in rendering a case bacteriologically negative, which was unfortunate in view of the fact that Maltese cases were to a large extent lepromatous. Some primary and secondary resistance developed to sulphones, mostly associated with poor compliance.

June 1972 – <u>Multi drug treatment ("MDT") started in Malta based on Freerksen's Malta Project</u>[32] All patients were treated with Rifampicin 600mg & 2 tablets Isoprodian (isoniazide 75mg prothionamide 75mg and Dapsone 50mg) for 2 years initially. Rifampicin is bactericidal and at follow-up 20 years later there were only 2 relapses due to non-compliance; out of a total of 237 cases that completed the MDT course. The period of treatment was determined by the clinical and bacteriological response. Split skin smears and biopsies were taken from numerous sites. Many patients had been on Dapsone for long periods prior to MDT. Bacteriologically negative patients were treated for 5 months. .The average duration of treatment was 24 months (2 to 172mths). Post-treatment surveillance was on average 12.26 years (0- 19 years).[33] After 2 to 3 months the patients began to feel better, their eyebrows began to return, muscles felt stronger, ulcers healed, and eyes improved. This had a tremendously positive effect on the patients.[34]

Dr S.K. Noordeen Director of WHO's Leprosy Elimination Programme at the time, stated that the Malta Project was a milestone in the fight against leprosy

Policy with regard to children

Except during the period of strict segregation children were not removed from their infectious relative. The youngest patient, in the 27 year progress report June 1972 – December 1999 following MDT, was 16 years old. [35]

Genetic Pre-disposition. Chromosome 6q25 has been linked with susceptibility to Leprosy "per se" and chromosome 10p13 to predispose to paucibacillary leprosy.[36]

1940 onwards - Health Education for Patients and Relatives. Public awareness is essential with an accent on early self presentation and case detection. As patients were being treated as Out Patients, education included hygiene and isolation in their own rooms with their own linen, towels, toothbrush etc. Financial aid to the families also encouraged the breadwinner to come forward. If the patient defaulted with follow-up attendances, financial aid ceased!. Job training, in permitted occupations, was provided.

Conclusions as to the factors favouring persistence of Leprosy in Malta until 2000.

1. Poor socioeconomic and insanitary conditions leading to poor host resistance.
2. The type of leprosy was 77% Lepromatous, the most infectious
3. Re-infection from outside Malta (see specific examples)
4. Taboo which militated against early detection and follow-up of contacts.
5. Antipathy to segregation, which caused general lack of co-operation.
6. No effective treatment until 1972, so no motivation to co-operate.
7. The long incubation period made the occurrence of cases unpredictable
8. Children were not removed from infectious mothers (except during segregation)
9. Genetic predisposition presumably explains why only certain members of the family succumbed to Leprosy.

Conclusions as to why Leprosy is now under control in Malta

1. Effective treatment in the form of Multiple Drug Therapy, which not only cured the patients but strongly motivated them to co-operate with their treatment and encourage their contacts to come forward. (See Table on Page 19 showing fall in incidence since the inception of MDT in 1972). This must be the most important factor.

2 Improved socioeconomic conditions and hygiene leading to improved host resistance.

3 Skilled professional personnel and bacteriological monitoring of progress and follow-up.

4 Health Education for patients and the population generally, especially with regard to early presentation, isolation and follow-up.

Bibliography

Paul Cassar - Medical History of Malta -Chap.20 p210 (1964- Wellcome Hist. Med Library)

Charles Savona- Ventura Outlines of Maltese Medical History (1997-Mid-Sea Books, Valletta, Malta)

J. Bugeja - Leprosy in Malta - p1347 (27/11/31 - Maltese Government Gazette)

Prof John Galea Chief Gov. MO and Dr Edgar Bonnici MD. Medical Superintendent of St Bartholomew's Leper Hospital, Malta - "Leprosy in Malta" (Leprosy Review 1957 VolXXVIII)

A.V.Laferla - British Malta (A.C.Aquilina. Malta)

Report by the Medical Secretary of BELRA (Leprosy Review Jan 1939 vol X no1)

Charles Savona-Ventura - History of Hansen's Disease in Malta (25/11/02 - www.geocities.com/hotsprings/2615/medhist/leprosy html)

Dr. Paul Gatt (present Leprologist in Malta) and Dr. George Depasquale (Leprologist 1972-89) kindly provided much valuable oral information and advice.

Principal Nursing Officer, Carmelo Abela provided first hand knowledge of Tal Ferha Estate.

ANNUAL INCIDENCE OF LEPROSY IN MALTA							
PERIOD:		ONE CALENDAR YEAR BY DATE OF NOTIFICATION					
DEFINITION:		NUMBER OF CONFIRMED CASES OF LEPROSY					
CRUDE RATIO:		NUMBER OF CONFIRMED CASES PER 10,000 OF POPULATION					
YEAR	CASES	POPU-LATION	CRUDE RATIO	YEAR	CASES	POPU-LATION	CRUDE RATIO
2000	1	391,700	0.03	1949	22	312,722	0.70
1999	0	378,500	0.00	1948	12	308,929	0.39
1998	0	377,000	0.00	1947	12	303,998	0.39
1997	1	375,000	0.03	1946	4	295,247	0.14
1996	0	373,000	0.00	1945	15	286,596	0.52
1995	0	376,335	0.00	1944	10	279,187	0.36
1994	0	366,451	0.00	1943	21	272,121	0.77
1993	1	366,431	0.03	1942	11	269,090	0.41
1992	1	362,977	0.03	1941	20	271,359	0.74
1991	0	359,543	0.00	1940	9	270,755	0.33
1990	0	355,910	0.00	1939	12	269,912	0.44
1989	3	352,430	0.09	1938	23	268,668	0.86
1988	2	349,014	0.06	1937	14	264,663	0.53
1987	5	345,636	0.14	1936	22	262,165	0.84
1986	3	343,334	0.09	1935	23	294,000	0.78
1985	4	340,907	0.12	1934	8	N/A	N/A
1984	0	338,276	0.00	1933	12	N/A	N/A
1983	1	335,169	0.03	1932	17	N/A	N/A
1982	4	331,859	0.12	1931	13	241,600	0.54
1981	1	328,375	0.03	1930	18	288,000	0.63
1980	2	325,721	0.06	1929	16	N/A	N/A
1979	2	322,535	0.06	1928	15	228,600	0.66
1978	2	318,320	0.06	1927	13	227,400	0.57
1977	1	315,466	0.03	1926	16	N/A	N/A
1976	5	311,150	0.16	1925	17	282,000	0.60
1975	7	306,551	0.23	1924	12	N/A	N/A
1974	5	301,892	0.17	1923	11	N/A	N/A
1973	8	302,219	0.26	1922	14	N/A	N/A
1972	4	303,114	0.13	1921	16	226,224	0.71
1971	6	303,161	0.20	1920	21	224,859	0.93
1970	7	302,820	0.23	1919	2	224,655	0.09
1969	8	302,486	0.26	1918	9	224,323	0.40
1968	8	302,340	0.26	1917	13	223,741	0.58
1967	12	302,218	0.40	1916	15	220,968	0.68
1966	10	318,109	0.31	1915	21	218,542	0.96
1965	16	316,440	0.51	1914	20	216,756	0.92
1964	11	320,620	0.34	1913	20	216,617	0.92
1963	13	326,130	0.40	1912	5	213,427	0.23
1962	10	329,326	0.30	1911	9	211,473	0.43
1961	14	329,763	0.42	1910	4	215,879	0.19
1960	9	328,938	0.27	1909	5	212,888	0.23
1959	15	327,218	0.46	1908	4	209,974	0.19
1958	15	323,667	0.46	1907	4	206,689	0.19
1957	21	319,957	0.66	1906	2	205,059	0.10
1956	19	316,239	0.60	1905	7	202,134	0.35
1955	13	313,955	0.41	1904	6	197,070	0.30
1954	10	315,952	0.32	1903	8	193,315	0.41
1953	11	320,613	0.34	1902	3	188,141	0.16
1952	14	316,764	0.44	1901	4	183,679	0.22
1951	5	312,646	0.16	1900	81	181,648	4.46
1950	11	312,447	0.35				

SOURCES: Maltese Health Information Systems Unit and Dr. Paul Gatt

Footnotes

1. Paul Cassar – Medical History of Malta Chapter 20 P.210 (Wellcome Historical Medical Library 1964)
2. Statistics for Europe – Encyclopaedia Britannica Statistics for Malta – Historical Demographical Data – University of Utrecht
3. Professor John Galea, Chief Government MO & Dr. Edgar Bonnici, Medical Superintendent of St, Bartholomew's Leper Hospital – "Leprosy in Malta" – Leprosy Review 1957
4. Paul Cassar - ibid
5. J. Bugeja, Malta Government Gazette Supplement 27/11/1931 P1347
6. J. Bugeja - ibid
7. Report of Committee to the Governor 1917 – Royal Malta Library ("RML") BR2 135
8. A.V. Laferla: British Malta 1977 Vol.2 P.48 – Publisher - Aquilina
9. A.V. Laferla - ibid
10. Government Gazette 1916 P. 373
11. Charles Savona-Ventura "Outlines of Maltese Medical History 1977 P.43 (Mid-Sea Books, Malta)
12. Charles Savona-Ventura - ibid
13. 1867 – Inquiry into Leprosy in the Colonies – Report by the RCP, London, RML B19 29
14. Committee appointed by the Governor 1868 to "Report on Distress"- RML Bp 5 74
15. Committee appointed by the Governor 1874 to "Inquire into & report upon the causes of recent increases in mortality in Malta" – RML BG 5 1
16. Malta Drainage 1883 – RML BL D 81
17. Dr. Diana J. Lockwood, , BMJ 2002 324/7352/1516-8
18. Ordinance VIII 1885 (17 September) Government Gazette
19. Dr. D.L. Leiker "On the epidemiology of Leprosy in Malta" Leprosy Review Supplement 3 38 - 41
20. Dr. Paul Gatt (present Leprologist in Malta) – verbal communication
21. Dr. Paul Gatt & Dr. George Depasquale (Leprologist 1972 -89) – "1972 – 1992 – 20 years after Initiation of Leprosy Eradication Programme in Malta".
22. Report on Health Conditions in Maltese Islands 1957 – Page 37 – Table XII and 1961 Table XII (Royal Malta Library).
23. Ordinance VII 1st March, 1893 "Measures passed by the Government for checking diseases commonly known as Leprosy" (Royal Malta Library CA4 2A Ext)
24. J. Bugeja, Malta Government Gazette, Supplement 17/11/1931
25. Charles Savona-Ventura, "History of Hansen's Disease in Malta" see Bibliography
26. Government Gazette 1916 P373, 1917 P 895
27. J. Bugeja, ibid
28. Leprosy Review, January 1939
29. Report on Health Conditions of Maltese Islands 1964 (Royal Malta Library)
30. J. Bugeja, ibid
31. Professor John Galea, former Chief Government M.O.
32. Enno Freerksen, Magdalena Rosenfeld, George Depasquale, Edgar Bonnici, Paul Gatt "The Malta Project – A country which freed itself from leprosy – A 27 year progress (1972 - 1999) – Chemotherapy 2001 : 47 P 309 - 331
33. Dr. Paul Gatt & Dr. George Depasquale, ibid
34. Chemotherapy – 2001:47 P 327
35. Enno Freerksen et al, ibid
36. Nature Genetics Vol 33 No3 March 2003 Page 412 MTMira et al 1991

12. C. Savona-Ventura: Leprosy. In: *Contemporary Medicine in Malta [1798-1979]*. Publishers Enterprises Group Ltd, Malta, 2005, p.79-82

13. C. Savona-Ventura. Rużar Briffa's contribution to leprology. The Sunday Times [Malta], 26th January 2006, p.17

Rużar Briffa's contribution to leprology

From Dr Charles Savona-Ventura, MD, D.Sc.Med. (Warsaw), FRCOG (UK), Accr.Cert.Obs-Gyn (Leuven), MRCP (Ire), CLJ, OMLJ

THE FEATURE by Dr Mark A. Sammut (*The Sunday Times*, January 15) reminded readers of the literary contributions made by Dr Rużar Briffa, who can be rightly described as one of the pillars of Maltese literature and a central figure in the foundation of the *Għaqda tal-Malti – Università* in 1931.

Because of his gigantic contributions to Maltese literature, his medical contributions are very often forgotten and put aside. Dr Briffa was one of the leading torch-bearers in the control of leprosy in Malta.

After graduating in medicine from the University of Malta in 1931, he was awarded the Strachan Travelling Scholarship, enabling him to proceed to London Institute of Dermatology where he followed an academic and practical course in the pathology and bacteriology of skin diseases.

On his return to Malta in 1932, he was a junior doctor in the Skin Disease Section at the Floriana Central Hospital. In 1938, he was appointed Leprosy Control Officer and proceeded to the Calcutta School of Tropical Medicine where he obtained first-hand experience in the manifestation and treatment of leprosy.

As Leprosy Control Officer and visiting consultant to St Batholomew's Leprosarium (1944), he continuously strove to combat the disease in the Maltese Islands by improving the living conditions of the inmates at the leprosarium and introducing innovative treatment protocols soon after they became available. He also promoted the removal of compulsory segregation of lepers, a regulation finally abolished in 1953.

Throughout his career, he maintained professional integrity by visiting centres of excellence, like the *Reparto Dermo-Sifilopatico* in Catania in 1949, and attending refresher courses, such as the one in leprology and skin disease at the *Policlinico* of Rome. In 1950, he was appointed senior consultant in dermatology at the Central Hospital and lecturer in dermatology and leprology at the University – thus ensuring a clear understanding of the disease to future practitioners.

His contribution to the field of leprology in Malta was acknowledged posthumously in 1973 when the former St Bartholomew's Leprosarium was renamed *Sptar Rużar Briffa* (after 1980 converted into an extension of St Vincent de Paul Hospital). In 1988, he was conferred the *Pro Merito Melitense* decoration by the Sovereign Military Order of St John.

While it is fitting to remember Dr Briffa's contribution to Maltese literature, it is also fitting to acknowledge his significant contributions to leprology especially since his death anniversary comes so close to World Leprosy Day.

C. SAVONA-VENTURA
Għargħur.

14. Buttigieg GG, Micallef Stafrace K. The Order of St. John's Crusade against leprosy. *Sacra Militia*, 2008, 7:29-38.

15. Cooke P. Leprosy is still a modern Maltese problem. *The Sunday Times of Malta*. 9th March 2014, p.6

Leprosy is still a modern Maltese problem

Patrick Cooke

Feared and misunderstood since biblical times, few would know there are still more than 30 lepers living in the Maltese islands.

A National Statistics Office report on social protection published recently revealed that 36 people were paid "leprosy assistance" in 2012.

This non-contributory benefit is paid to any head of household who suffers from leprosy, also known as Hansen's disease, or who has a member in their household suffering from it.

The number of people receiving the €34.94 weekly allowance is slowly dwindling each year, with 57 individuals receiving it in 2007. This year just 32 qualified for assistance, the Social Solidarity Ministry said.

"There are still a number of old-time sufferers of Hansen's disease living in Malta. I emphasise these are non-infective cases," explained Charles Savona-Ventura.

Chev. Prof. Savona-Ventura is Grand Prior of the Grand Priory of the Maltese Islands of the Military and Hospitaller Order of St Lazarus of Jerusalem.

The priory has traditionally assisted lepers and still supports a number of ageing Maltese lepers living in the community.

There are no longer any lepers living in institutions.

A group of lepers were housed for a long time at St Bartholemew Leprosarum at St Vincent de Paul Hospital. Twenty-four were transferred to Hal Ferha Estate in 1974.

> "There are still a number of old-time sufferers of Hansen's disease living in Malta. I emphasise these are non-infective cases"

Hal Ferha closed down in 2001 when the only remaining case was transferred to St Vincent de Paul. The last institutionalised leper died several years ago.

There is a deep social stigma attached to leprosy because it can cause skin lesions and severe physical deformities, but modern-day treatments mean the disease is treatable and non-infective.

Leprosy primarily affects the peripheral nerves, skin, upper respiratory tract, eyes, and nasal passages.

Though widely assumed to be spread via the respiratory system through nasal droplets, broken skin is also a possibility.

The Grand Priory has an NGO affiliate called the Raoul Follereau Foundation (Malta) – the Order of Charity, which collects funds to support the worldwide fight against the disease.

Despite leprosy being curable, it is still a disabling scourge in third world countries because treatment is not readily available, Chev. Prof. Savona-Ventura said.

The Order of Charity circulates an annual newsletter among its 1,600 members and issues posters and circulars to all parish churches and church schools.

In 2013, the Order distributed almost €15,000 to around 20 associations worldwide who work with lepers.

Anyone wishing to assist the Order of Charity in its fight against leprosy can send donations together with their name and address to: Order of Charity, Catholic Institute, Floriana.

H: Leprosy Eradication Project of Malta

16. A. Agius-Ferrante, G. Depasquale, E. Bonnici, C. Paris, W. Grima: The leprosy eradication-project of Malta. *Z Tropenmed Parasitol.*, 1973, 24:Suppl 1:p.49-52.

17. A. Agius-Ferrante: First Investigation. *2. Intern Leprakongress For-schungsinstitut Borstel*, vol. 1 (suppl.), 1973

18. G. Depasquale: The Leprosy Eradication Programme of Malta. *Leprosy Review*, 1975, 46 (Suppl. 2):p.215-217

19. G. Depasquale: Rifampicin and isoprodian in combination in the treatment of leprosy. *Leprosy Review*, 1975, 46 (Suppl. 2):p.179-180

20. E. Freerksen, M. Rosenfeld: Leprosy eradication project of Malta. First published report after 5 years running. *Chemotherapy*, 1977, 23(5):p.356-386.

21. E. Freerksen, M. Rosenfeld, E. Bonnici, G. Depasquale, H. Kruger-Thiemir: Combined therapy in leprosy. Background and findings. *Chaemotherapy*, 1978, 24:187-201

> Abstract: This report is based on data obtained from 64 lepromatous cases. Despite many years of DDS monotherapy, the homogenates from biopsies of these patients revealed 10(4) or more bacteria. From the beginning of combination therapy with synergistic-acting substances

(rifampicin + isoprodian (INH + PTH + DDS) the logarithms of the number of bacteria in the homogenates decreased, both during treatment period and during treatment-free observation period (Figs. 3--8). During the whole time biopsies were taken almost monthly. A considerable regression of the bacterial mass or even "negativity" could be observed within a relatively short time. Once started, the process of reduction of bacteria continued also after termination of therapy. To be able to evaluate a medication, therapy-free observation periods (for a minimum of 5 years) are indispensable.

22. G. Depasquale, E. Bonnici: *Leprosy eradication project of Malta – Report after 6 years running.* Lecture given at the XI International Leprosy Congress in Mexico, 1978.

23. W.H. Jopling, M.J. Ridley, E. Bonnici, G. Depasquale: A follow-up investigation of the Malta-Project. *Leprosy Review*, 1984, 55(3):p.247-253.

24. D.L. Leiker: First assessment of the Malta Leprosy Eradication Project. *Leprosy Review*, 1986, 57 (Suppl 3):p.42-46.

25. D.L. Leiker: On the epidemiology of leprosy in Malta. *Leprosy Review*, 1986, 57 Suppl 3:p.38-41.

26. G. Depasquale: The Malta experience. Isoprodian-rifampicin combination treatment for leprosy. *Leprosy Review*, 1986, 57 (Suppl. 3):p.29-37.

27. W.H. Jopling: A report on two follow-up investigations of the Malta-Project. *Leprosy Review*, 1986, 57 (Suppl 3):p.47-52.

28. D. Vella Briffa: 'Eradication' of leprosy from Malta. *Leprosy Review*, 1987, 58(1):p.87-89.

29. E. Freerksen, M. Rosenfeld, G. Despasquale, E. Bonnici: [The Malta project (a program for the eradication of leprosy)]. *Acta Leprol.*, 1988, 6(5):p.7-46.

30. E. Freerksen, M. Rosenfeld, G. Depasquale, E. Bonnici, P. Gatt: The Malta Project--a country freed itself of leprosy. A 27-year progress study (1972-1999) of the first successful eradication of leprosy. *Chemotherapy*, 2001, 47(5):p.309-331

   Abstract: The successful conclusion of the first leprosy eradication program carried out with combination therapy is reported. This program started in Malta in June 1972. It was based on extensive experimental and clinical studies and was formally concluded on 31 December 1999. No new infections occurred after the start of this 27-year progress report. The youngest patient was 16, and the eldest 83 years old. Of the total of 261 cases in the project, 201 had already received pretreatment [mainly with diaminodiphenylsulfone (DDS)] at the start. Sixty-one cases had no pretreatment. These were predominantly elderly patients who were late in deciding to have treatment. The very long follow-up period totalling 27 years was consistently maintained in order to be able to refute all potential objections empirically, e.g. with regard to relapses at a late stage. Besides the overall symptoms which are typical for the broad picture of leprosy, the involvement of the eyes was very striking (at least 50%). The therapeutic effect was of very rapid onset in these cases without surgery. Rifampicin (RMP) + isoniazid + prothionamide + DDS (trade name Isoprodian-RMP) was used as medication in a fixed combination. This fixed combination had already proved to be highly effective in the treatments during the course of the project, surprising therapy results (including lifesaving effects) were also noticed in other diseases.

Maltese Legislation

1. *Notizie della Sacra Infermeria*. Rome, 1725 (English translation: E.E. Hume. Medical work of the Knight Hospitallers of Saint John of Jerusalem. John Hopkins Press, Baltimore, 1940, 137-148)

   - Records the allowances given to victims of lepers in the community during Hospitaller times.

   "The Ordinary and Extraordinary Charities of the *Sacra Infermeria*. ... In the first place, as has already been mentioned, it is the duty of the *Prodomi* to provide daily allowances to all the poor, lame, leprous, and scrofulous people, and other invalids, which amount at the present time to 100 scudi the month."

2. Ordinance XX of 1919: To make provisions with respect to the disease commonly known as leprosy. The Lepers Ordinance Chapter 73 of the Revised Edition. Eventually amended by Act. XV of 1929, Ord. XXV of 1939, Ord. XVI of 1942, amended by Government Notice 174 of 1949 and mostly repealed by Act XI of 1953. Amended by Act LVIII of 1974, Legal Notice 148 of 1975, Act VIII of 1990, Act V of 2007, and Legal Notice 346 of 2008.

SUBSIDIARY LEGISLATION 45.01

LEPERS REGULATIONS

27th June, 1939

GOVERNMENT NOTICE 285 of 1939, as amended by Government Notice 174 of 1949 and Act LVIII of 1974.

1. The title of these Regulations is Lepers Regulations. — *Title.*

2. There shall be a medical officer in charge of each Leper Hospital hereinafter referred to as the "hospital". — *Medical officer. Amended by: G.N. 174 of 1949.*

3. Each hospital shall consist of two divisions, male and female. No communication shall be allowed between the patients of either division, or with persons outside the hospital, except as is permitted by these Regulations. — *Two divisions.*

4.* There shall be an established diet for the patients which may be altered or added to by the medical officer in charge of the Hospital when the condition of any individual patient so requires. Such alterations or additions shall be noted in the diet book of the institution against the name of the patient concerned. — *Established diet.*

5. Patients detained in the hospital may have food provided for them by the relatives and friends, but no articles of food or drink shall be introduced if, in the opinion of the medical officer in charge of the hospital, such articles are objectionable on grounds of health or discipline. — *Provision of food by relatives.*

6. Patients may use their own clothing, undergarments and bed linen, provided that they have a quantity which, in the opinion of the medical officer in charge of the hospital, is sufficient to ensure proper cleanliness. Otherwise all articles of clothing and bedding and all undergarments shall be supplied by the hospital. — *Clothing, undergarments and bed linen.*

7. The washing of all articles used in the hospital shall be done in the hospital laundry. No article used by the patients shall be taken out of the hospital. — *Laundry.*

8. All letters from patients shall be delivered to the medical officer in charge of the hospital for disinfection before they are despatched to their destination. — *Letters.*

9. Patients may be visited by their relatives and friends on such days and at such hours as may be fixed the Chief Government Medical Officer, and under such conditions as the medical officer in charge of the hospital shall consider necessary. — *Visiting days and hours.*

10. Patients who are dangerously ill may be seen by their relatives or friends on any day and at any hours during the daytime, on application to the medical officer in charge of the hospital. — *Dangerously ill patients.*

---

*The original regulation 3 has been omitted, under the Statute Law Revision Act, 1980, in view of the fact that it referred to provisions contained in article 6 of the Ordinance, which article has been repealed.

Permission to patients to leave the hospital for temporary periods.	11. The Chief Government Medical Officer may grant permission to patients to leave the hospital for temporary periods under such conditions as he may consider necessary to impose in each case.
Leprosy Board.	12. The Leprosy Board shall visit the hospital every twelve months to examine patients and attend to other professional matters with the medical officer in charge.
Discharging patients from hospital. *Amended by: G.N. 174 of 1949.*	13. The medical officer in charge of the hospital shall inform the Leprosy Board of the case of any patient whose condition has, in his opinion, improved to an extent that might justify his conditional discharge from the hospital. The Board shall examine the patient and submit a report to the Chief Government Medical Officer on the state of the disease in the patient and shall make such recommendations as it may think fit relative to the patient's conditional discharge from the hospital.

Discharged patients.
*Amended by:
G.N. 174 of 1949.*

14. All patients discharged shall conform to the following conditions:

(a) they shall inform the Chief Government Medical Officer through the medical officer in charge of the hospital of the address at which they intend to reside on discharge and of any subsequent change of address;

(b) they shall present themselves to the Leprosy Board for examination once every six months, or more often if so required by the Board;

(c) they shall not engage in any trade, business, occupation or work of the following nature -

   (i) any trade or business connected with the supply, preparation or distribution of food, drink, drugs, medicine or tobacco in any form;
   (ii) laundry work;
   (iii) tailoring;
   (iv) domestic service;
   (v) nursing;
   (vi) midwifery;
   (vii) hairdressing;
   (viii) itinerant hawking;

Treatment out of hospital.

15. Patients who are not removed to, but are to be treated out of the hospital shall present themselves for treatment at such place and time as may be ordered by the Chief Government Medical Officer. All such patients shall present themselves to the Leprosy Board for examination once every six months, or more often if so required by the Board. Nursing mothers shall not be allowed to nurse their babies.

Patient who has been conditionally discharged.
*Amended by:
G.N. 174 of 1949.
LVIII.1974.68*

16. In the event of any person who has been conditionally discharged from the hospital developing contagious manifestations of leprosy, the Board, through the Chief Government Medical Officer, shall inform the President of Malta who may revoke the order for the conditional discharge of any such person and order his removal to the hospital. In the event of any patient undergoing

treatment out of the hospital developing contagious manifestations of leprosy, the medial officer in charge of the hospital or any other medical practitioner who becomes cognisant of the fact shall at once inform the Leprosy Board, and the Board, after examination of the patient, shall through the Chief Government Medical Officer inform the President of Malta, who may order the removal of the patient to the hospital.

17. Patients who, in the opinion of the medical officer in charge, are able to contribute some assistance to the service of the hospital or to perform agricultural, needle or other work, may be so employed in return for extra comforts or a small monthly gratuity to be fixed by the Chief Government Medical Officer.

Patients able to contribute assistance.

18. The members of a household where a case of leprosy has occurred may be subjected from time to time to medical examination.

Members of household.

19. Any patient who contravenes these Regulations or the rules of the hospital; or who disobeys the orders of the medical officer in charge of the hospital; or who creates any disturbance; or who uses obscene or profane language; or who insults, or reviles, by word or deed, an officer or servant of the hospital or another patient; or who commits any nuisance in any part of the hospital; or who damages or destroys government property or articles belonging to other patients, shall be liable to any or all of the following punishments as may be decided by the Chief Government Medical Officer:

Contravention of these Regulations. Amended by: G.N. 174 of 1949.

(a) suspensions of leave of absence;

(b) stoppage of the allowance of money for tobacco, or stoppage of wine, dessert or any other article of food;

(c) deprivation of a drive in the country.

The period of any of the above punishments shall no,t in any case, exceed one month. More serious offences shall be dealt with according to law.

CHAPTER 45

LEPERS ORDINANCE

To make provisions with respect to the Disease commonly known as Leprosy.

(19th September, 1919)*

Enacted by ORDINANCE XX of 1919, as amended by: Act XV of 1929; Ordinances: XXV of 1939 and XVI of 1942; Acts: XXXIX of 1948 and XI of 1953; Legal Notice 46 of 1965; Act LVIII of 1974; Legal Notice 148 of 1975; Acts VIII of 1990 and V of 2007; and Legal Notice 346 of 2008.

1. The short title of this Ordinance is the Lepers Ordinance. — *Short title.*

2. (1) No leper coming from any place outside Malta shall land at any of the ports of Malta.

(2) The provision of subarticle (1) shall not apply to persons born in Malta.

(3) The master or other person in charge of any vessel who suffers or permits or fails to prevent the landing from such vessel at any such port of any person whom he knows or has reasonable grounds to believe to be a leper shall, on conviction, be liable to the punishments established for contraventions.

Alien lepers prohibited from landing in Malta. Amended by: XI. 1953.3; L.N. 46 of 1965 LVIII. 1974.68; L.N. 148 of 1975; VIII. 1990.3; V. 2007.25; L.N. 346 of 2008.

(4) Every leper so landing as aforesaid may by warrant of the President of Malta be committed to a hospital designated therein and there detained for such time as may be fixed in the warrant.

Measures to be taken in case of landing.

(5) Every leper so landing as aforesaid may be brought before a magistrate of the Courts of Magistrates, who may examine such leper and any other witness on oath, concerning the place from which such leper came to Malta, and may cause such leper to be removed to such place in such manner as the President of Malta may direct.

(6) The reasonable cost of such inquiry and removal shall be borne and paid by the master or other person in charge of the vessel by which such leper was brought to Malta, or by whose act or default such leper was permitted to land.

(7) Such cost shall be recoverable as a civil debt due to the Government by proceedings before the Civil Court, First Hall.

(8) For the purposes of the preceding provisions of this section the decision whether a person is a leper shall rest with the Administrative Review Tribunal established in terms of article 5 of the Administrative Justice Act and the provision of this Act shall apply to such an appeal.

Cap. 490.

(9) The said board shall respect and apply the principles of good administrative behaviour laid down in article 3 of the Administrative Justice Act.

Observance of the principles of good administrative behaviour. Cap. 490.

---

*See Proclamation No. XVII of 1919.

SOCIAL SECURITY [CAP. 318]
CHAPTER 318 SOCIAL SECURITY ACT

To establish a scheme of social security and to consolidate with amendments existing provisions concerning the payment of social insurance benefits, pensions and allowances, social and medical assistance, non-contributory pensions and the payment of social insurance contributions by employees, employers, self-employed and the State.

1st January, 1987 ACT X of 1987, as amended by Acts XX of 1987, XIV of 1988, XVI of 1989, VIII, XVI of 1990, XIII of 1991, VIII of 1992, XXIV of 1993, XXV of 1994, XXVII of 1995, XXI of 1996, XVI, XXII of 1997, VII of 1998, II of 1999; Legal Notices 56, 84 of 1999, 10 of 2000; Act XI of 2000; Legal Notice 21 of 2001; Act VI of 2001; Legal Notices 4, 422 of 2002; Acts II of 2002, XI of 2003; Legal Notice 436 of 2003; Acts II of 2004, III, XIII of 2005, II, VI, XIX of 2006; Legal Notices 100, 101 of 2006, 62, 318, 424 of 2007; Act XXXII of 2007; Legal Notices 105, 149 of 2008; Act II of 2009; Legal Notices 143 of 2009, 437 of 2010; Act IV of 2011; Legal Notices 330, 455 of 2011; Acts I, V of 2012; Legal Notices 117, 218, 342 of 2012; Act IX of 2013; Legal Notices 355 of 2013, 62, 79 of 2014; Acts XII, XXXVI of 2014, XIII, XXXIX of 2015; Legal Notices 123, 258, 302 of 2015; Acts XV, XXVII of 2016; Legal Notices 309, 337 of 2016, XVI of 2017 and Legal Notices 6 of 2018, 44 of 2018 and Act VII of 2018 and Legal Notice 195 of 2018.

21. (1) Subject to the provisions of this Act, a person who is the head of household shall be entitled to Leprosy Assistance if he shows to the satisfaction of the Director that he or any member of his household is receiving treatment for leprosy. *Leprosy Assistance.*

(2) Where such head of household has been continuously in receipt of Leprosy Assistance since the 14th April, 1975 at the rate applicable on that date, he shall continue to receive such assistance at that rate, as long as he is not entitled to a higher rate of Leprosy Assistance in terms of the provisions of this Act.

(3) Sub-article (2) shall not apply where there has been a change of circumstances in the household.

NINTH SCHEDULE
[Article 25]

Amended by: XIV. 1988.19.
Substituted by: XVI. 1990.55; XIII. 1991.47; VIII. 1992.45; XXVII. 1995.17. XXI. 1996.63. XXII. 1997.11; L.N. 56 of 1999; L.N. 84 of 1999; L.N. 10 of 2000; L.N. 21 of 2001; L.N. 4 of 2002; L.N. 422 of 2002; L.N. 436 of 2003; L.N. 100 of 2006; L.N. 101 of 2006; L.N. 318 of 2007; L.N. 424 of 2007; L.N. 149 of 2008; L.N. 143 of 2009; L.N. 437 of 2010; L.N. 330 of 2011; L.N. 342 of 2012; L.N. 62 of 2014; L.N. 123 of 2015; L.N. 309 of 2016; L.N. 6 of 2018; L.N.195 of 2018.

Type of Assistance Weekly Rate
3. Leprosy Assistance:
    (i) in respect of the head of household who is a leper   €36.11
    (ii) in respect of any other member of the household who is a leper and not gainfully occupied:
        (a) if under 16 years of age   €21.79
        (b) if 16 years of age or over   €36.11
    (iii) in respect of any other member of the household who is not gainfully occupied   €21.79

www.ingramcontent.com/pod-product-compliance
Lightning Source LLC
Chambersburg PA
CBHW081810220526
45466CB00006B/2243